A New You Your 14-Day Makeover

by Gloria Richards

VENTURA BOOKS
New York City

Printed in the United States
All Rights Reserved

© COVER PHOTO BY ALEX GOTFRYD

CONTENTS

INTRODUCTION

How do I know my crash course in fitness and beauty will work for you? Because it worked for me. I'm not one of those beautiful people who have been perfect from the cradle, nor have I always had the good habits that keep a human face and body in top condition. I learned—the hard way—that fitness is for life. I never wanted to be a size 14 again, and I saw that the only way to prevent it was to change my ways—for good. I know about the needs of working women, mothers, couples—I know because I've been there.

My 14-day program wasn't designed in 14 days. Over the years, I've tried to distill the essential features of a real makeover—body, face, hair, clothes, the works—into a system that helps people fast, before they get discouraged. I think I can promise you that if you follow my program, and if you continue to maintain the good habits it will give you when the 14 days are over, the result really will be a "new" you.

The Basics

To be perfectly clear, my book is not for people who can go to Swiss clinics or spend half of every day in a beauty salon. *My* life hasn't been like that, and neither are the lives of most women. Most of us don't have an English Nanny at home to watch the toddlers while we attend class. My diets are diets that real people can follow—they don't require you to eat caviar and prime rib three times a day. And my makeup and hair programs don't come from people who work only on the faces of movie stars and models; they come from my experience and the experience of hundreds of women. And they work. They work for people with ordinary faces, bodies, lifestyles, and bankbooks. My system can help you lift your face and figure out of the ordinary into the striking, the beautiful, the classy. And all you need is this book, plus a firm commitment to really, this time, *do* it.

As a woman with a lifelong commitment to fitness and beauty, I've seen all the techniques, treatments, gimmicks and fads, and I can tell you which ones are sound and which ones are a waste of time and money. I wish, for my sake and yours, that every rash promise of every beauty promoter were true. But they aren't, and you might as well know it. Once in a while, a diet or treatment is actually dangerous. More often, it's just wasteful for you and easy money for the promoter. When you're through with my course, you'll be able to tell the difference. I'll tell you the truth about:

> Hair color
> Sun bathing
> Cellulite
> Jogging
> Plastic surgery
> Wrinkles
> Makeup
> Hair—excess and otherwise
> Diets, all kinds

And that's not all. I'll tell you how to put it all together in the kind of crash course women keep begging for.

To really take advantage of my program, you have to read the whole book. Otherwise, you won't understand why you have to do things the way I've spelled them out, and you might be tempted to cheat. Learn the basics first, then proceed to your personal makeover. At the back of the book, I've put some of the questions most frequently asked about the program and about health and beauty generally. The answers you'll find are the answers I've discovered from working with people and listening to their needs. Take a look at the outline of our 14-day program, but don't start on it until you've studied the information in the early chapters. Remember, I didn't trip over this system on the sidewalk—it's been refined through thousands of hours of experience. Just relax, read, and put yourself in my hands.

THE 14 - Day System

Day 1: The Beginning. First of all, unless you're underweight, you'll start your diet. A reducing diet is part of the program, and you aren't really following the course if you aren't trying to do something about your weight. Second, grooming. Third, exercise. You'll be reminded about the Big Three every day. Finally, there's that special thing you do for yourself each day to promote lasting beauty and attractiveness. Today, it's the Hair Cut, because there's no better instant morale booster than a session with a really talented trimmer.

Day 2: Hair—the Other Kind. This day's devoted to hair you don't want, how to take it off and keep it off: the pros and cons of various methods of hair removal, and which ones you can do yourself.

Day 3: Facials, masques, deep cleaning, all the down-under care your skin has to have to look great when the makeup's on. You'll experiment this day to find the right skin-care routine for your skin's special requirements.

Day 4: The Bath. Yes, it's for getting clean, but that's not the half of it. Wise women consider the bath part therapy session, part fountain of youth. Do you know how to use this precious time to its fullest advantage?

Day 5: Hair Conditioning. All about all of them—the new chemical miracles and the age-old but still good oil treatments, kelp baths, milk rinses, and more. Try them all today, pick what you like for long-term hair care.

Day 6: Hands and Feet. The pedicure, the manicure,

and most of all, Fingernails. Here's how you can duplicate those expensive and time-consuming salon treatments at home. Very relaxing, too.

Day 7: Here's the rub. Body massages you can do for yourself or someone else, and vice versa. Plus, body moisturizing, a must for those, like you, who are taking off excess pounds.

Day 8: Into the second week, and now you'll start studying how to decorate your clean, soft, and somewhat smaller body. This day's devoted to the Wardrobe Game—it may be the first time you spent three hours in a closet, but you'll love it.

Day 9: The Hair Routine. How to plan a program of care that's right for you—without spending all your time on your hair. Your new haircut is one week old, and you can learn a lot from seeing what's happened in that time.

Day 10: Makeup Essentials. What's available, and what it can do for you. This day, you'll figure out what you need in your makeup kit, and what you can leave on the shelves.

Day 11: The eyes have it. But do yours? Maybe your eye makeup routine needs to be re-thought. If so, this is the time.

Day 12: Face shaping: the delicate art of contouring to minimize faults and maximize good looks. Takes some practice, but worth the time once you learn how.

Day 13: All about lips: how to reshape your mouth, what kinds of lip color are best for you, plus the necessary tools.

Day 14: Lifetime Makeup Routine: It's time to put it all together in a program you can carry on without giving up your job, your children, or your life. In other words, how to condense everything you've learned into the legendary (but possible) ten-minute everyday makeup routine.

Chapter I: Basic Facts About Hair

A very rich woman once said that she spent more time and money on her hair than she did on clothes. The reason? "If your hair looks super, it doesn't matter what you're wearing. But it doesn't work the other way around." Beautiful hair beautifully cared for is the single most important feature of a great beauty. And the wonderful part is that almost everyone can have beautiful hair. It isn't like a beautiful nose, for which you either have to be very lucky in the genetic lottery or spend a bundle on cosmetic surgery. It isn't like beautiful clothes, which take a stylist's eye and a good deal of money. It isn't even like a beautiful body, which, depending on how out of shape you are, takes a lot of time and effort.

For all the above reasons, we start with hair. You *can* and you will have a beautiful body and a beautiful face, but you can get beautiful hair even faster. It's all a matter of know-how and technique. What you have to know is what hair really is, and what kind yours is. Then you can move to treating your problems and playing up your assets.

Most hair is built in three layers. There's the medulla, or inner layer, the cortex, in the middle, where the pigmentation is located, and the cuticle, or outer horny layer. Most hair treatments act on the cuticle. Some, like permanent waves and hair color, penetrate the outer layer to work their changes, though they make no changes on the color of your hair as it grows, as anybody who has ever suffered the "dark roots" stage can testify.

There are no products that work on the medulla, and indeed, some hair, the very fine, flyaway kind, may lack the inner layer altogether.

As for the texture of your hair—whether it's coarse or fine, straight or curly—that's determined by your genes. It used to be thought that people with curly hair had curly follicles, but that's not so. It's the hair that grows out of those follicles that curls or doesn't. Nothing will permanently straighten curly hair or curl straight hair. A "permanent" is only as permanent as the hair it works on. Chemical treatments have no effect on what's going on under the skin as each hair is growing out of its follicle and up toward the surface of your scalp. That's why we'll never be done fussing with our hair—because the hair just won't be done with growing.

When you hear people speak of "nourishing" the hair, they mean one of two very different things. Hair can be nourished—with good food, the right amount of exercise and sleep—in short, with a healthy routine. Since hair is almost entirely protein, you do have to have adequate protein in your diet to produce beautiful hair. But, of course, you have to have adequate protein for just about every other body system, too, or more vital ones than hair will begin to fail if you don't. Beyond that, there's not much known about the effects of diet on hair. Since hair is actually dead by the time it emerges from your scalp, most of the good your diet does for your hair takes place at the invisible stage. All the same, you can't have shiny, healthy hair without a healthy you.

The other sense in which hair can be "nourished" is from the outside. This is the same sort of thing as "nourishing" the wood of your fine furniture with the right oils and polishes. The furniture isn't really alive, nor is your hair. But both can reap the benefits in appearance that come from proper treatment. And both can be damaged by improper treatment. Luckily, however, the resemblance ends here. Furniture, once dried, bleached, or burned, won't grow out. But no matter how rough you've been to your hair, it's only the old hair—the hair that's already sprung from its follicles and appeared on your head—that you have damaged. There's always new growth, in natural if not perfect condition, waiting to take the place of the old. A damaged chair may have to be thrown out, but there's always hope for damaged hair.

How long your hair grows, and how long it takes a permanent or other lasting treatment to grow out, depends on many things, most heavily on heredity. The average life of a human hair is between two and five years. Since hair grows about six inches in a year, that means that the upper limit of hair length is about 30 inches, or something under three feet. Sometimes, you'll see women—lucky ladies—with hair even longer than that, and it means that their hair—every hair on their heads—has a longer-than-average "head life." This explains why some people can't grow below-the-knee locks, not even when they try, while others can hardly keep up with their flowing tresses. It used to be thought that only women could grow really long hair, and it was even explained in an old textbook on hair that this difference between the sexes demonstrated the greater need of the "fair sex" for protection. Presumably, back in the cave days, the long hair of the women kept the rain off—or something. Actually, many young men can, if they're so inclined, grow hair longer than many women. It is true, however, that men tend to lose their hair earlier and more completely than women, so that while a fifty-year-old woman might easily have waist-length hair, a fifty-year-old man most likely could not. Maybe that's why, though hair is sexy in either men or women, it has been and still is the "crowning glory" of a woman. Women just have a better shot at getting and keeping beautiful hair.

The reason that men go bald more often than women (who, alas, can also be troubled with hair loss and even baldness) seems to have something to do with androgen, the male hormone. In men, androgen produces the characteristic male pattern baldness. You know, first his forehead lengthens, then suddenly there's no hair on top at all, just a fringe around the edges like Brother Sebastian. This sort of thing almost never happens to women, though male pattern baldness affects (or afflicts) more than half of all men. If your man is afraid of going bald, tell him to take a look at his father, grandfather, uncles, and so forth. If they have male pattern baldness, chances are he will, too. There's really nothing to be done about it short of hair transplants, which are expensive, itchy, if not downright painful, and often don't really do much good. (Think of Frank Sinatra and William Proxmire, two prominent people who made no secret of the fact that they'd had hair transplants. Both are still—or once again—baldish gentlemen with only slightly more hair on the tops of their heads than they would have had if they'd left well enough alone.)

Women, too, can look to family history for hints about how age and hormones will affect their hair. If your mother or grandmother or great-aunt has experienced marked thinning of the hair as she grew older, perhaps—just perhaps—you will, too. It all depends on whose genes you got for that particular characteristic. The kind of thinning that affects women is usually spread all over the head, not concentrated in certain areas as it is for men. A more common problem than baldness for older women is slowed growth. That's one reason that even women who *always* wore their hair long, often cut it when they reach middle age. It just takes too long to replace one of those long hairs, and the result is thinner, less luxurious hair—older looking long than short.

There are, of course, health factors that can contribute to abnormal hair loss in both men and women. But these are relatively rare and always the sort of thing one notices, such as prolonged high fever, surgery, the recent birth of a child. (That last one's for women only.) As in all abnormal conditions, the solution is to correct the underlying health problem, and the hair problem will take care of itself. Hair loss after pregnancy is really just compensation for the abnormal, though nice, hair retention *during* pregnancy. When all your post-partum symptoms subside, you should have just about as much hair as before you got pregnant. There are also local diseases of the scalp that can cause falling hair and temporary baldness, but, once again, these abnormalities are accompanied by other symptoms, such as severe itching, scabs, and so on, so you really can't confuse them with the quiet, inexorable loss of hair that comes from just being you and getting a little older. Naturally, if you suspect any disease—either organic or one of the skin and scalp—consult a physician.

Once in a while, a severe shock, either to the body or mind, can cause hair loss or graying, though I've never heard of a case where the hair really "turned white overnight." If you narrowly miss being tossed off a cliff by an escaped lunatic, you might experience some symptoms in your hair, as well as elsewhere. But it takes a *real* shock, and not just your daughter's announcement that she doesn't want to attend your alma mater after all. (If your hair turns gray after that one, you can figure it was going to turn gray anyway.)

Tricks and Treatments for Baldness

Though women aren't likely to fall for some of the hairy schemes perpetrated on unsuspecting folks in the name of treatment for baldness, they might have husbands or fathers or lovers or brothers who will. To be complete then, let's just discuss some of these schemes, and why you should advise your men to stay away from them.

Hair Weaving

This rather odd practice involves hooking strands of

the recipients own hair—two or three strands at a time—under the skin of the scalp to make a sort of permanent toupee. Only it isn't really permanent—it only lasts until the strands cause infection in the skin around them and fall out. This unsavory practice can lead to horrendous-looking scalp lesions, and will always end, eventually, in the same broad plane of baldness you had at the beginning. Reputable doctors won't do this, and why would you want to see anyone else?

Massage, scalp treatments and the like.

If baldness is due to a genuine disease of the scalp, then of course, treatment will help. But male pattern baldness happens to people with perfectly healthy skin and scalp, and no amount of rubbing the top of your head with sweet-smelling oils (or foul-smelling ones, either) will change the destiny of your head. Lots of men have spent lots of money having a specialist in tonsorial flim flam shine lights on their heads, give them tar shampoos, and wrap their heads in hot towels. It may feel good, for all I know, but it won't make your hair grow. All of these "specialists," by the way, will unabashedly claim that they definitely can make hair grow, and even trot out "proof," in the form of friends who say they were bald as eggs before the treatment. Often, they will even make their extravagant claims to consumer protection officials and reporters, though they have also been known to close up shop very fast under threat of real investigation. Enough said?

Hair transplants

These are for real, and are done by legitimate medical men. In the long run, the results are often disappointing, and there is some pain associated with the process, but if you go to a reputable doctor, you won't end up with a head that's one big infection. Unless you're a movie star, wouldn't it be easier and safer just to face up to the fact that you're going bald?

Tension baldness

This isn't really a disease, but it isn't hereditary, either. It's the kind of baldness you bring on yourself when you "tear out your hair," or "snatch yourself bald." Most cases today don't arise from fury, however, but from mechanical devices such as tight rollers, rubber bands, or unusual headgear. Luckily, most of us have turned away from fashions such as the pony tail and French twist, and hot rollers have made it pretty much a thing of the past to sleep all night on brush-filled torture rods. But if you still pull your hair tight for any reason, consider that you might be pulling it out, at the same time. If you find your hair coming out in clumps when you take down your elaborate hairdo, or if you've been getting thin patches since you started wearing your ultra-tension nightcap, better cut it out.

Dandruff

As long as we're discussing un-health, we should mention a very common scalp problem that sells tons and tons of dandruff shampoo a year and has probably bothered every one of us at one time or another. To begin with, all of us have flaking scalps. It's in the nature of the skin up there to shed old cells as the new ones mature. In a healthy situation, the shedding is gradual and the flakes stay small, so they aren't noticed on the shoulders of your navy blue suit or sexy black sweater. But when the cells don't shed in a normal way, they pile up on the scalp and shed in *big* flakes, the kind that everybody notices. This condition, if it gets serious, can also cause itchy scalp and even infection.

If your dandruff is mild, it may be that you just need to encourage circulation in your scalp a little to promote normal function. A regular scalp massage will do it, or maybe just some regular brushing with a gentle, natural-bristle brush. Dandruff shampoos do work, but they are stronger medicine than the manufacturers would have us believe. If you decide to use one, you should be aware that it may cause damage to your eyes if you get it in the eye itself. There's a warning on the bottles, of course, but not everybody takes those things seriously. Please, do.

Sometimes, dandruff is a seasonal problem, coming on in the winter when everything, including the growth and sloughing off of your skin cells, has slowed down. If you start using a dandruff shampoo, don't let the habit blind you to the fact that your condition has cleared up. And don't keep using the dandruff shampoo past the time when you need it. Contrary to what the advertising may tell you, it isn't really the best all-purpose treatment for healthy hair. On the other hand, some people have more trouble with dandruff in the summer, when their oil glands are likely to be over-active, and producing too much of the sebum, or scalp-oil that all of us have on the surface skin of the head. This condition causes the flakes to flake off faster than normal, until you feel as though it were snowing from your head. What's worse, the oil causes the little flakes to stick together into big flakes, and you know how unpleasant that is. In either case, be watchful, and cancel treatment when the condition is gone.

If none of the usual home remedies work for you, and you still consider your dandruff a serious problem, it's time to see a skin doctor. It's just possible that you really do have a scalp disease, and not just an exaggeration of a normal condition. Sometimes, skin disease of a more general type masquerades as "dandruff." During the course of your dandruff difficulties, incidentally, it's best to avoid wearing dark clothes, and it's definitely a good idea to keep your scalp and hair extra-clean. If you suspect your dandruff is caused by a dry scalp, use a conditioner or even a little bit of olive oil or baby oil in your hair to restore moisture.

Healthy Hair

Most people don't have any real diseases, not even dandruff. Does that mean you haven't got any hair problems? You know better. Healthy hair is just a beginning on the way to beautiful hair, but it's the essential first step. How do you know if your hair is in good shape? Well, if you haven't been treating or mistreating it, it probably is. Hair that has been permanent waved, permanently colored, straightened, or bleached is tender hair, and it needs extra special treatment. That goes for hair that's been baked under the summer sun and bathed in chlorinated swimming pools, too, of which more later.

If you haven't been abusing your hair, here's a good test to find out whether it's in good shape: Pull out one of your hairs, (ouch!) and look at it closely. If it's about the same diameter as a piece of ordinary thread, it's pretty thick as hair usually goes. If it's very much thinner than thread, you have fine hair. Another good comparison is to hold your hair up against the hairs of several good friends. (Casual acquaintances won't let you take hairs without a fight, so please don't try.) Is yours the thinnest? The thickest? Just about average? This informal comparison can tell you a lot about the texture of your hair. Next, take the hair firmly by both ends and stretch it. If it has good elasticity, the hair should stretch about twenty percent of its length without breaking.

If your hair can pass the stretch test, it's in good condition, no matter how coarse or fine. You can't really do much about the texture of your hair, but healthy hair of any type has its own special appeal.

Suppose, though, that your hair won't pass the stretch test? That means that there's something you've been doing that you ought to stop, or something you ought to be doing that you haven't. The most common abuses of hair these days are over-bleaching, over-heating, and overprocessing. For some hair, once is enough with the bleach bottle or the curling iron to dull and dry the hair shaft. Other kinds of hair—usually the heavier, thicker textures—can take quite a lot of processing before they get brittle and dull. Only you and your experience can determine how much is too much for your hair, but if you've been tinting, bleaching, permanent curling or straightening, and your hair won't stretch, perhaps you should consider giving up the process.

If you can't get along without your tint or your permanent—and there are good reasons why women say they can't—you'll have to start on a program of conditioning. Analine dyes and the caustic solutions in permanents are very hard on the outer layer of the hair, the cuticle. When the cuticle is in good condition, all the little layers lie flat, and reflect the light to give you that marvelous shine that everyone wants to have and to see in beautiful hair. After chemicals have been applied, however, the layers of the cuticle get roughed up—they don't form a flat surface and they don't shine. One advantage to this—and this is of special interest to those of us with baby-fine hair—is that it makes the individual hairs thicker, and it makes your whole crop of hair look fuller, fluffier, just *more*. Unfortunately, those who most need body and bulk, the ones with fine hair, are usually the ones whose hair suffers most from overprocessing.

To counteract the effects of too much processing or too much sun, condition, condition, condition. Buy a conditioning shampoo, a conditioning rinse, a deep conditioner. You might want to try a hot-oil cap from time to time. During your 14-Day Makeover, you'll learn about all kinds of hair conditioners, and you'll experiment to find what's right. But I can tell you now that if your hair is suffering from processing blues, you have to start right away on a religiously regular program of restoration and repair. The longer you've been abusing your hair (and the longer your hair is, by the way), the more important it is.

Even hair that has never seen the open mouth of a haircoloring bottle may not be able to pass the stretch test. If that's the case with you, your hair may just be structurally weak. Now that you know it, you'll know how to take care of your problem hair. First of all, don't start processing. Your hair can't take it. Yes, I know, you have such fine hair that if you don't have a permanent it seems to just lie there. But better lying there than breaking off an inch from the scalp. The answer for you is probably a short cut that will fluff up with a minimum of setting or heat, and, like your overprocessed sister, you should condition, condition, condition. For special occasions, you might consider learning how to work magic with switches and hairpieces. Actresses and models all know how, no matter what their hair types. Why not you? (Fine hair, it turns out, often completely lacks the inner layer of the normal three-part hair construction. That's why it's so fine, and that's why it can lack the elastic strength of thicker hair.)

Dry hair

Dry hair is the hair that grows out of a dry scalp. That means that your sebaceous glands are underactive—they don't secrete enough oil to keep your hair shiny and bright. If you have thick hair (large diameter hairs) and especially if you have thick hairs and lots of hair (more follicles per area), dryness may not be such a problem. It means you don't have to shampoo as often as others, maybe once a week or even less. As long as the dryness isn't causing a scalp condition, or due to chemical treatment of the hair, moderation in shampooing plus regular conditioning should be all you need.

Suppose, though, that your hair is fine or thin or both? Dryness combined with those circumstances can create flyaway hair with a vengeance. Sometimes, in the winter especially, people with this kind of hair feel like (or look like) they've just been through the clothes dryer. Again, you could start by being grateful for small favors. Dryness means you don't have to wash your hair every night, a time-consuming preoccupation of your oily-haired counterparts. Depending on your face shape, you might want to adopt a hairstyle that's firmly anchored, such as a relaxed, loose twist. Nothing, actually, is lovelier than long, shiny, fine hair, and you can only get away with it if your hair is at least a bit on the dry side. Can you imagine having to wash a yard and a half of hair every night? Another solution can be the good short cut, but remember, you have to maintain it even more rigorously than most, or you'll start to look like you've been through Dr. Frankenstein's generator again.

Oily Hair

The other extreme from dry hair means the other problem with the oil glands of the scalp—they're working overtime. This is a common problem with teens and women in their twenties, and sometimes they don't notice when the condition of their hair changes. They go right on using harsh detergent shampoos and using them often, even after the need is gone. These days, those kinds of shampoos aren't necessary for anybody. Not with the recent advances in cosmetic chemistry. Now you can get a gentle, conditioning shampoo, especially formulated for hair that needs to be washed often—even every day—but doesn't need to be turned into a haystack in the process. If you do wash often, one of these shampoos can be the best investment you ever made in your hair. They cost a little more, but they're worth it.

Creme rinses are usually out for oily-haired types, but there are now instant conditioners that rinse out, just like creme rinses, and don't leave a greasy film (causing the "limpies," or the "droopies".) Another expedient as old, at least, as your grandmother, is the vinegar or lemon-juice rinse. These aren't so good for body, but they're terrific for shine—work best if your hair's both oily and thick. As for oily, *thin* hair, the chief problem is keeping it ultra-clean, so it won't look plastered to the head. That usually means daily shampoos, which, in their turn, mean daily quick conditionings plus regular deep-down treatments. Most hairdressers advise that people with this hair type keep it short—no longer than chin-length, and layered a little to promote the full look.

Shampoos

How to pick the right shampoo from that imposing array on your druggist's shelves? First, read the labels. This may be a bit intimidating at first, but you'll see, once your eyes get used to the difference between laurel sulfate and *laureth* sulfate, that many of the shampoos have the same ingredients, regardless of price. If you like to use a nationally advertised brand of baby shampoo, for instance, take a look at the cheaper, house brand of baby shampoo next time you shop. Does the label read like a photocopy? Then buy whichever's cheaper. Like other products, the house brands are often made in the very same factory by the very same process as the famous brands. On the other hand, if your favorite conditioning shampoo has sixteen ingredients while the cheap brand has five, stick with your favorite. You can bet it has more sophisticated chemistry behind it, even if you can't pronounce all the names.

What about pH-balance in a shampoo? The answer is that it's probably a good idea to use hair-care products (and skin-care products, too) that come close to the natural pH of the skin—neither too acid nor too alkaline. Nobody is exactly sure just what having the acid-base balance disturbed does to the skin or hair, but it stands to reason that you should tamper with nature as little as you have to. Strong soaps and detergents are more alkaline than the skin (pH about 5), and so almost every manufacturer now tries for acid-balance in its shampoos. You don't have to think about the right pH very much, because most hair-care products have it. But don't be alarmed if you've been washing your hair with dishwashing soap, at least not on account of your hair. The skin restores its acidity very soon after washing. But now that you know better, stop using the dish soap, especially since nobody has gone to any trouble to run tests on it to see it it's harmful to *eyes,* as cosmetic companies do with their shampoos. Note: if any shampoo or hair-care product makes your skin break out or itch or turn red, discontinue it at once. This is true even if you've been using the substance for years. Allergic sensitivity can develop at any time—not just the first time you use a product.

Styling

As we've said, the single most beautiful thing about a woman can and should be hair. And the single most important factor in beautiful hair is how you wear it. That's true no matter what shape your hair is in, though the better its condition, the better it will look in the right style. Nevertheless, a great haircut can conceal a multitude of sins, at least while you're busy correcting the damage.

What determines the hairstyle that's right for you? Everything: your lifestyle, your schedule, your hair type, your face shape, your complexion, your age, your manual dexterity, just everything. Sometimes, it takes years of adult living before we find just the right way to wear our hair for a minimum of fuss and a maximum of good looks. But there is one person who can make all this a lot easier, and that's the right hair stylist. Today, the cut is all in professional hair care, far more important than the set, say, which most of us haven't had for years. We want hairstyles that don't have to be set, pinched, sprayed or pinned. Lots of us won't (or can't) even wield a blow dryer in the service of chic. But we want to look good, all the same, and it's all left up to the cut.

Now, for a spot of bad news. It turns out that in haircuts, price is really a good indicator of quality. That means that cut-rate cuts usually aren't worth it. Because a really good precision haircut has become the be-all and end-all of hair styling, people who know their business can command high prices, and they do. There's virtually no such thing as "getting it wholesale," unless you happen to be married to your city's top stylist. Hair stylists sell a service, not a product. *They* can't get it cheaper, so they don't sell it cheaper. There's just no way around it: if you want the best haircut, you're going to have to pay top price.

If you really can't afford the going rate for a good haircut, there are some ways to save. To keep you as a regular client, your hairdresser will probably be glad to cooperate. If your salon will let you, wash your hair at home before you go. That way, you only have to pay for the cut, not the shampoo or rinse or whatever. Another way of cutting corners is to do without the blow-drying, though some salons won't give you any price break on this. But it doesn't hurt to ask. (If it's winter, don't forget to bring a hat to cover your wet head. Hospitals are far more expensive than hairdressers.) You'll lose time by shampooing first and then rushing home to style your hair yourself, but you will undoubtedly save money in the bargain. Don't however, try to save by not tipping your hair stylist. There's no using trusting your hair to someone who has a grudge against you for your penny-pinching. The only time you don't have to tip is in a owner-operated salon. If your stylist is also the proprietor, he or she doesn't need that little extra to pad the salary.

I do not recommend beauty colleges or barber schools for precision haircutting. You have to remember that many salons run schools to raise money, and there's no guarantee that any of their graduates will be the same high quality as the people they hire to work "up front." Naturally, if the training is good, some of the graduates will be good. But there's no way in the world for you, the customer, to tell from looking at them which is which. True, the schools are much cheaper than the salons, but then so is having your head shaved.

Finding a Stylist

So how to get a regular hairdresser who can make your hair look right every time? The best strategy is just to shop around among the salons in your area with high-class reputations. As with doctors or dentists, ask your friends. Ask especially those friends who always seem to have great-looking hair. (But beware the natural beauty. There are some women whose hair is so thick and shiny and gorgeous that a two-year-old with a pair of baby scissors could make it look good. Ask friends who say they have some hair problems, too.) If you do your shopping in quality establishments, you'll never get a really lousy cut, and eventually, you'll find Julie or Pierre or Mr. Bud who can bring out the stunning you.

If you have to check out salons without recommendations, here are a few suggestions. The trendier salons are usually the better ones. Whether the latest fashion is green-and-white wallpaper and lots of plants, or silver-and-glass and lots of loud rock music, the hippest *looking* salon is usually staffed with the best and most fashion-conscious cutters. It doesn't matter if you can't stand rock music or if green-and-white makes you ill. You probably do want the best haircut you can find, and that's probably where you'll find it. Watch out for old-fashioned looking shops where all the customers seem to be little old ladies with blue beehives. They might just give you a blue beehive, too.

When you go to a new stylist, or even to one you've used before, don't go with a head completely empty of ideas. The stylist will have some suggestions, but you should have suggestions, too. The truth is, nobody knows your hair better than you do. You may seem to have very fine, flyaway hair that couldn't hold a set if the rollers were left in all night. But perhaps you know from a lifetime of experience with your hair that it takes a set very quickly—the result of just a trace of natural curl that you always brush out when you dry. It could take a stylist many sessions and the memory of a pachyderm to know that little fact about your particular head of hair, but you could clue him in, in a matter of seconds. And once you're sure of something about your hair, don't be talked out of it. If you know you have a cowlick on the right side and your hair *cannot* be parted there, don't let the stylist part it. Both of you will be dissatisfied if you get what you're dead set against.

On the other hand, be prepared to listen to what the stylist has to say, especially if your own notions of what you want are still fairly vague. You may want a short look, but not be sure if that means a Mia Farrow cut or just shoulder-length instead of hair you can sit on. The stylist can tell you which will work best for your hair, your life, your face. If you're looking for a style to last the rest of your life, say so. But if you want to experiment, say that, too. Some stylists will try to talk you into changing your look every few months just like the models do. If consistency is your thing, say so. And if your stylist keeps bugging you about getting the new "fringy" look or chopping your hair off an inch from the roots, get a different stylist. (A good hairdresser will always put the will of the customer first, even if he or she thinks you're wrong. We want to be advised, not forced).

THE CUT

Once the initial decisions have been made—Short? Long? Curly? Layered?—the cut can begin. What you should be doing while Evelyn or Jack is cutting is watching as closely as you can. There's a strong temptation in a beauty salon to relax, daydream, stare at the other clients and try to imagine what they do for a living. But you're going to have to work with this hair that's being cut every single day until your next haircut, and knowing exactly what's been done to it can help make your job a lot easier.

First, watch to see that Jack knows what he's doing. A

good cutter will carefully section the hair, pinning other sections out of the way of the one he's working on. If Jack seems to be going at your head in a series of random snips, he's not the man you want to make a regular arrangement with. Is he smoking, gazing around, chatting to the guy in the next chair? (These days, it's just as likely to be a guy as a woman.) Something's not right. Jack should be concentrating on your hair. Let him have a cigarette, if he has to, on his own time. About this business of conversation: I know it's very common for hairdressers to talk to each other, visit with the clients, sing, or whatever. I prefer that mine doesn't, at least not much. Of course, I always exchange pleasantries, and give quick consideration to the news or the weather or whatever. But in general, I want my expensive haircutter to be paying attention to my expensive haircut. Far be it from me to get his mind off the track. Besides, they take longer when they're talking.

If you're watching what's going on, you can tell the stylist that you don't think the sides are quite even, that you've spotted a stray long hair, or—and this is most important—that you think he's taken off enough, that you don't want it any shorter than that. If you're not watching, you might have a negative surprise when you come out of your daydream to discover that you look a lot like the dog does when she's just come back from her annual summer shearing. Don't be afraid to offer suggestions and even criticisms during the cutting as well as before it starts.

The Style

When the cut is over, your stylist will probably use a blow-dryer to finish your style. If at no other time, you have to pay attention during this operation, that is if you want what you do at home to come anywhere close to what the stylist does. (Or even if you don't. If you don't like how your style comes out, you can style it differently by avoiding what the stylist did.) Perhaps you think you aren't very good with the blower. Here's how to get better. Pay close attention to just what the hairdresser does. You can't exactly duplicate what's done at the salon, because you'll be working on your own head instead of behind it. But much of our clumsiness with the necessary electrical gadgets of the now styles comes not from natural klutziness, but from not having the faintest idea what to do once we move the little switch from "off" to "on."

Often, it you don't like the way the style seems to be shaping up, ("What are those little wings on the sides?") the stylist can change course while the hair's still a bit damp. Most hairdressers have told me that they'd rather deal with a client who's alert and sure of her opinion, even if she does make them change things a little. "I like the interaction," says one. "It keeps me alert, keeps me doing my best work." That sounds like the kid of thing we all want to foster, doesn't it? Although we offer specific tips on how to use all the electric appliances during your 14-Day Makeover Course, you'll find that what you read about come alive when you watch an expert in action. And don't be shy about asking questions. Some people seem to regard the hairdresser as they do the doctor: they don't want to inquire too deeply into the "mysteries." In my opinion, you'd be better off if you asked *both* of them plenty of questions.

A caveat about electricity. All the electric appliances that make hairstyling so much easier and quicker these days work by heating up the hair. All that heat can damage the cuticle, and therefore can dull your hair's shine and de-condition it. But it doesn't have to happen if you compensate by more moisturizing and careful care. Just one more reason we've devoted a whole day in your makeover program to conditioning. Today, as never before, hair protection is just as important as style.

Chapter II:
Hair Coloring and Treatment

So you think you want to color your hair. Or you already have colored your hair. Either way, chances are you don't have all the facts. Because nobody does, not yet. Is coloring bad for your hair? Is it bad for you? There are arguments both ways. Research into some questions about haircoloring has hardly begun, while others have been under intensive scrutiny in the laboratories of the cosmetic companies for years.

As with all products and practices that aren't at least a hundred years old, there are questions about haircoloring. The same goes for any strong chemicals used on the skin. (Don't forget that what's under your crop of luxurious tresses *is* skin, just like what covers all the rest of you.) Many chemical substances penetrate the skin, get picked up by the blood, and are circulated to distant parts of the body. Solutions used in haircolorings and permanent waves are no exceptions. In fact, because the circulation system of the head is especially good, chemicals applied to the head are more likely to get into general circulation than those applied in other places.

So what? you may be saying, and the answer must be that nobody knows what just yet. Some tests have suggested that dyes derived from coal tar—which includes all the permanent and semi-permanent products for haircoloring now on the market—can cause tumors in laboratory animals. But we know by now that what happens in the laboratory is related only in a very complex way to what happens outside. Researchers still don't understand if what happens to laboratory animals has any real relevance to what happens to women (or men) who color their hair. We have seen one such study, the Surgeon General's report on smoking, gain general acceptance, forcing even tobacco industry people to concede that smoking can lead to lung cancer and other diseases. We have seen another study—that of cyclamates and saccharine—fail to have meaningful results for humans. The verdict simply isn't in yet on hair colorings. I do think that reasonable people should be willing to give up any practice that is really *proved* to be harmful to health: I know I will, if evidence forces me to think that my haircolor is really dangerous. So far, I'm not convinced.

As for other physical side effects, such as skin swelling, rashes, and burns, careful patch testing every time you use a coloring or permanent wave solution will prevent those. Why every time? Because, as I've said before, sensitivity can develop—seemingly out of the blue—at any time. Remember, that all of these solutions, even the semi-permanent colorings, are either strongly alkaline or contain metal salts, both kinds of substances known to cause allergic reactions in some people. Actually, the number of reactions is small, but don't you become one of them. Take the time to take the patch test recommended in every package of home hair treatment.

Now, about the psychological side effects—which is why we really color our hair in the first place. There's no denying the lift it can give to a woman's appearance and her spirits to go from drab, mousey, graying or just boring to terrific. And there's no doubt whatever that hair color can do that for you. Some of the drawbacks have already been mentioned. Here are some others: If you don't like your new color, and it's permanent, you'll have to wrestle with months of "growing pains," as the hair slowly returns to its natural color. Of course, you can always put a new color over the one you don't like, but if it's haircoloring in general you've decided against, there's nothing to do but wait. And then there are the touch-ups. For most of us, that's every four to six weeks, and it rolls around faster than you'd ever suppose. It's one thing to spend the afternoon messing with your hair because you feel like it, and quite another to do it because you have to—the roots are starting to show. There are other problems, too—faded color, and the fragile condition of your hair once you've used a strong chemical on it. Besides all that, if you use a shampoo-in coloring, you're treating most of your hair to another chemical bath every time you touch up.

On the positive side, there's the beauty of most of our new haircolor products, particularly when they're used properly. There truly has been a revolution in cosmetic chemistry in our lives, and I've seen colored hair that was as lovely, as soft, as natural-looking as any child's. Though your hair really is in tender condition after you've colored it, it doesn't have to look like it or feel like it—not with the absolute battery of conditioners at our disposal. And bright, shiny color just makes most of us look and feel better about ourselves. There's no better way to get a younger look, a more alive and vigorous look than haircolor. For many of us—and I include myself—it's worth the trouble and expense. (I prefer professional salon coloring, and I recommend it if you have the money. Professionals don't get careless and make the mistakes we tend to make at home—you know, "Oh, the phone rang while I was timing my toner, and I completely forgot to check the clock.") Besides, my stylist knows how to mix shades in the most impressive way—I'd swear this is the color my hair was when I was ten.

If you're ready for haircoloring, if you think the benefits outweigh the detractions, it's time for my primer of types.

Temporary Colors

These are the ones that you rinse or shampoo in, rinse or shampoo out. They're almost always completely gone after the first shampoo, certainly after the second. Unfortunately, they also run away if you go swimming, sweat a lot, or even walk in the rain. Some people find that a lot of the color applied the night before stays on the pillow when they get up in the morning. The best use of temporary color rinses is to try out a slightly different shade to see if you'd like to have it more permanently. Notice that I said a *slightly* different shade. Don't expect any startling new haircolor from temporary rinses—they just can't deliver.

The reason for the completely temporary and mild nature of temporary haircolor rinses is that they don't penetrate past the outer layer of the hair shaft the way permanent or even semi-permanent colorings do. They just coat the outside of each hair with pigment. It only sticks as long as the hair stays dry. Naturally, this is the least damaging of all color treatments. Temporary color leaves the hair essentially as it found it once you wash it out. Another plus: though temporary color rinses won't change your hair's color much, they can give more body to fine, limp hair. It just stands to reason that a hair with a coating of color will be thicker and stand away from the other hairs. And these rinses won't damage your hair, they really won't. That means you can use them after each and every shampoo if you want to.

Semi-Permanent Colors

Most of us today lead such active lives that having to stay out of the rain, and not *sweat,* for heaven's sake, simply won't fit in with our lifestyles. How can you jog, how can you dance, how can you play tennis without perspiring? I'll bet even Jackie Onassis does. What that means for those of us who want to color our hair is that we need something that won't come off so easily as temporary rinses do. The next step is semi-permanent hair colorings, the kind that say on the package that they last through four to six shampoos. (They used to say four to six weeks, until cosmetic copywriters discovered that most women wash their hair considerably more often than once a week. It's not the time that determines how long these products last, it's how often they're subjected to shampooing.)

The good thing about these middle-of-the-road products is that they can give stronger coverage than temporary rinses without peroxide or other strongly alkaline chemicals. The bad part is that if, like me, you wash your hair every day, they only last a week or less, making these semi-permanents pretty darn temporary. Furthermore, although they'll cover a few gray hairs very gracefully, if you have a lot of gray—say, more than twenty percent—they won't do the job. Although semi-permanent colors do get inside the outermost layer of the hair, every time you shampoo the hair swells and lets some of the molecules of coloring agent back out. In a few weeks, (or a few shampoos, whichever comes first), you're back where you started. Many women prefer these products, even though they have to be applied more often than permanent analine dyes, because they don't leave any marked growth line—they fade gradually as you shampoo, and because they do effectively cover a small amount of grey without changing the color of the rest or your hair—if you pick the shade closest to your own.

Permanent Colors

These are the products that come the closest to what we really want when we dye our hair—a new color, for good. Of course, as I said before, it isn't for good, but only until the new growth begins to show. The chemist who discovers how to dye the hair in the follicle (without damaging anything) will make more money than Rockefeller. But don't hold your breath until that discovery is announced.

Basically, there are three kinds of permanent colorings.

There are the metal salts, the kinds of colorings that wash in gradually but stay in permanently, and claim to duplicate your natural color. The big problem with these products is that the metal compounds are really quite unstable. A lot of sun, a swimming pool, or just time may turn your metallic-dyed hair bright orange, purple, or green. I've known men (most users are men, because they like the gradual nature of the color change) who suffered terrific embarrassment from suddenly clown-like hair. And you can't cover a metallic-dye mistake with an analine-dye antidote, because the peroxide in the latter will cause your already stressed hair to snap off at the roots. Men, luckily for my friends, can get away with a crew cut much more easily than women, for whom I strongly recommend some other product.

Next, there are the natural, vegetable dyes, the ones that have been with us at least since Cleopatra's time. The ancient Egyptians loved henna, for example, and used it extensively to accent their shining black hair. Henna, the most popular of the natural dyes, and the only one that I know of that is widely available in salons, is also the safest thing you can use to color your hair. Since you can, if you're so inclined, even *eat* henna, you can be pretty sure it won't hurt you even if it penetrates the scalp and gets into the bloodstream. Like other coloring agents, henna makes the hair look thicker. Unlike analine dyes without conditioners, it also makes the hair look and feel healthier, shinier, silkier.

What, you're asking, are the drawbacks? Well, for one thing henna is incredibly messy, at least in the effective forms. It dyes your fingernails, too, and seems more reluctant to come out of them even than the hair. Henna isn't too good at covering lots of gray, mostly because the colors on gray or white hair look too stark—either orange-red, dark brown, or black-black. The best strategy is to have your henna treatments in a salon —this may be more important with henna than with any other coloring agent. Actually, very few home preparations are available, and those that are seem to be inferior in coloring power to what salons can get.

Finally, there are the permanent colorings that use peroxide, either shampoo-in types or creme types, salon or home. These include the one-step tints as well as the two-step bleach-and-tone products for making dark hair much lighter. As you are most likely aware, these are by far the most popular coloring agents, and the ones that cosmetic chemists are working on night and day to improve. I think the reason for their overwhelming popularity is twofold: first, the colors you get with this method of coloring really are the truest, the most natural, and the most varied. Second, they're as permanent as they can be—they never wash or rub off, as even henna and metal-salt dyes have been known to do.

Analine dyes are also the harshest on your hair, especially if you use the two-step processes. Since the hair shaft is penetrated by both the coloring agent and the peroxide, the cuticle is considerably roughened. Without conditioning, your hair would have that straw-like look that used to be associated with (pardon the term) bleached blondes. But modern chemistry has put lots of conditioners right into the coloring agent, and you can buy lots more to use between colorings. Some analine dyes actually leave the hair softer and shinier than it was when it hadn't been treated at all—at least on initial application they do. Some of us have found to our disappointment that after the next shampoo, however, the hair felt a bit stripped and tangled. That's why each shampoo for color-treated hair must also be a conditioning session. Your hair has undergone some weakening, there's no way around it. To compensate, you must condition every time you wash, like a fanatic.

Hair colored by any of the "tints" or "toners" included in this method can be permanent waved (as hennaed hair cannot). Many hairdressers, however, caution against too many processes. As the famous Mr. Kenneth says, "I don't believe in doing everything to the hair. You have to make a choice." My experience—yes, I tried it once, against advice—is that a permanent makes the colored hair brittle, and can fade the color, too. The next time you color, you may find your hair so porous that it admits more color than it should, and you don't get that great shade you were so happy with before. All in all, it seems to be the best idea to choose one or the other, or else get ready to spend a lot of time in the hairdresser's chair, having the damage fixed. And if you're even contemplating a dual-processing extravaganza, by all means have each step done in a salon. Tell your colorist and stylist exactly what you have in mind before *any* process is begun.

About color fading. It seems to happen with the best of products if you live the way I do—out in the sun, swishing through the pool, shampooing all the time. I've come to think that my kind of hair— very fine is the name of the kind—may be more subject to color fading than thicker hair, but it seems to happen, and the only answer is a fresh coloring job. I have my hair tinted at a salon, so that my colorist can see just how much fading has taken place and correct it. It seems to be worse in the summer, as you might expect. If your hair has a lot of red in it, even if it's just undertones, you may find that the shade you pick comes up ruddier on your hair. Drabbing solutions are available to correct this in your home hair tints and toners, and salon colorists have such things on hand. Don't forget to mention your hair's tendency to go red before the colorist begins his or her work. It'll save you time and grief at the other end of the process.

Which Process for You?

The haircoloring product you need depends on what you expect to get from coloring your hair. If you just want to try some shade for a party, then temporary rinses are what you want. Remember, though, they can't make you blond for a night, not unless you're blond to begin with. What they can do is add extra sparkle to your own hair color, maybe cover a few stray gray hairs—temporarily.

Perhaps you'd like to cover those gray hairs on a regular basis, but don't want to run the risk of having your color drain off into the swimming pool. On the other hand, you don't want peroxide, either. After all, what if you change your mind? If that sounds like you, you're the one the cosmeticians had in mind when they invented the semi-permanent colors. Remember the two big drawbacks—if you shampoo often, semi-permanent colors will only last a week or so and (this may be the reason so many women go on to the permanent colorings) they're really just as messy and time-consuming as the more lasting varieties. I wish I could tell you there's a product you could just splash on and rinse off in the shower that would cover gray and bring the life back to your haircolor, but there just isn't—not yet. But don't think the cosmetic companies aren't aware of that. You can be sure they're working on it.

Now: the permanent dyes. First of all, I'd say stay away from the metallic solutions—too risky. After that, there's natural permanent tinting, usually henna. This can be the perfect solution for some women, but not for all. It's best to have henna put on in a salon, which means a certain amount of regular expense. And—here's the real drawback—the range of colors is really fairly narrow. You can have natural henna, which is no color at all, but adds body and shine to the color you've already got. After that, your basic choices are to go redder, browner, or blacker. And the effects are somewhat upredictable, even when the job is professionally done. You may come out much redder, for instance, than you'd expected. An ameliorating factor is that henna fades gradually—like the semi-permanent colors, only slower. And henna won't cover more than about 20 percent gray hair, at least not in a shade that blends in with the rest. There's always a danger in trying to cover a head of hair that's really two different colors—usually gray toward the front and darker toward the back—that you'll end up looking like one of those flashy two-toned cars our fathers used to drive. The danger is increased with henna.

Now, we come to the product everybody really thinks of first when they think of haircoloring. Well, really it's two separate processes: the one-step tint and the two-step tint. Both are really trickier than they seem, though home hair colors have improved drastically in the last few years, especially with the advent of the "shampoo-in" products. Still, there are matters like the greater absorbency of gray hair, hair near the ends, and hair nearest the face. Directions will always tell you to do these areas last, but that's pretty hard to do if you're trying to use the haircoloring just as you would your shampoo. Generally speaking, you'll still get much better results if you have a professional colorist do the job. I think the shampoo-in home colors work best for women with almost no gray to cover, and look most natural when they're close to your natural shade. Yes, you can make rather dramatic alterations with just one step, but the farther away you get from your own color, the more it's hard to predict the exact shade. And you might experience an unpleasant surprise the second or third time you use the same product. It acts differently on already-tinted hair, which yours will be after the initial application. Another unpleasant surprise that can happen with either the one-step or two-step processes in hair breakage. Hair made brittle from too much solution can snap off, usually near the scalp. If there's much of this, it gives you thinner, not thicker hair, plus the disconcerting feeling that you're going bald. (You're really not, at least not for ever.)

Two-step processing is what you need if you want to go from dark (darker than dishwater) to blond. Step one is the bleaching where the dark color is lifted out of your hair by a peroxide solution that penetrates to the cortex and changes your natural color. Step two is the new color—shades of blond are almost infinite. You really can go as light as you want with two-step processing, but it's hard on your hair. And the lighter you have to go, the more the solution weakens hair. I don't think, personally, that two-step blonding should be done on very fine hair. It's just too much of an assault on hair that isn't very tough to begin with. And retouching is so much more risky with two-step blonders. You can't just do the whole process over and over on your whole head of hair the way you can with the shampoo-in colorings. Not only will your hair finally break off in odd places, but you'll get funny shadings where the new job overlaps the old. These effects are increased with fine hair.

I guess which process you choose depends on just how important the exact results are to you. If you really have your heart set on being a blond, and you're fully aware of what the upkeep will mean in terms of time and money, go ahead. As they say, you only have one life. But if you're just flirting with the notion of "wouldn't it be fun," or, "I have to do something about those gray hairs anyway, why not just go blond," think again. It's really too much trouble to be undertaken carelessly. (Women whose hair has already gone completely gray or white are in a different position, since they probably don't have to undergo the bleaching step. This is often a good solution for the older woman who doesn't want to stay gray but whose skin color is no longer suited to the dark hair she had as a girl.)

Light touches

As you must know by now, there are more ways to put a little light in your hair than just to do the whole thing blond. Frosting has been with us for some time, and is often a perfect solution for the woman who wants to hide the fact she's getting gray without committing herself to a completely new color. It's also good for just putting a little snap into drab hair—and it works, if carefully done, on dark hair as well as light. You can have subtle effects or more dramatic coloring, all with the same process. And you can touch up pretty much when you feel like it. Since the whole head isn't colored, dark roots are much less apparent. These days, frosting has been joined by tipping, streaking, face-framing, and hair painting. They're all basically the same idea: highlight the hair with little streaks of blond. I think it looks wonderful on young women whose hair was on the light side anyway, or to highlight warm brown hair. It's not my favorite solution to graying hair, because the contrast between the natural darkening that usually happens as hair begins to gray and the lightening necessary in frosting or streaking can begin to seem harsh. But that's just my personal opinion. For some women, it's the ideal answer.

If you want to put just a few touches of lightness in your hair—the way the sun might have done if you'd spent the summer at the beach instead of at the office, I think one of the home hair painting kits can work very well. But you have to have the patience to do it slowly— just a few hairs at a time. For those with darker hair, tortoise-shell painting kits are available. They give your hair light brown highlights instead of blond, and they really do look better on brunettes. For anything more extensive, including traditional frosting with the cap and all, see your colorist.

Some streaking jobs only require a lightener—the first step in traditional two-step blonding. It's left on long enough to bleach the strands to the desired lightness, then neutralized. More extensive highlighting usually means two-process treatment, but remember, it's not working on all your hair, so you usually don't have to worry about the haystack effect. Best of all, streaking and frosting grows out with grace, especially if you've used a restrained hand to begin with.

A final thought: peroxide, though poisonous to drink, has been used as a surface antispectic for a long time, and is not thought to harmfully penetrate the skin. It's unlikely, therefore that lightening strands of hair, especially if you don't need a toner, will cause harmful side effects somewhere else in your body. This is not so clearly true of the shampoo-in or one-step tints. Peroxide is harder on your hair, though, and the blonder you want to get the more you'll have to use.

Permanent Waves and Straighteners

Essentially, these are the same, even though the effects they aim at are opposite. A solution is used to break the bonds in the cortex that hold your hair in its straight (or curly) shape. Then the hair is re-shaped, either on rollers or by stretching it straight, and the solution neutralized. Your hair now has the shape it took on in the re-shaping process. Is all this hard on the hair? Of course. Is it worth it? It all depends. In the past, the big problem with permanent curling was frizz. Lately, permanent wave solutions have been gentled, altered, controlled. All the same, a minute too long before neutralizing or the wrong solution for your kind of hair can give you a permanent case of the frizzies. The home permanent is still a risky business. (Even the so-called "body" waves can make your hair too curly and make hair care more, not less, time-consuming.)

The trouble with hair straightening is the opposite—it doesn't last. Straight at first, your hair seems to emem*ber its curly old self and strains to resume its old shape. You end up setting your hair all the time to make it smooth, just as before.

I think both permanent curling and permanent straightening work best with styles that are regularly set. If you're prepared to go that route, you can get some spectacular effects. But if you're hoping for hair that exactly duplicates the naturally curly or the naturally straight—hair that needs no fussing-with to achieve its best look; I think you're out of luck. Even the "natural" frizzy perms— "just run your fingers through them" don't really work like naturally curly hair. You can never get that close-cropped curly look, for instance, because you need a certain length of hair to wind around the permanent waving rods, and subsequent to the permanent, what's close to the scalp isn't the curly part but the straight hair growing out. The grow-out difficulty also affects straightened hair, though not so drastically if the hair is long. Sheer weight will straighten hair near the scalp—for a while.

If you tint your hair or feel it takes chemical solutions easily, be sure to tell your stylist before permanent curling or straightening begins. There are different permanents, and some will suit the condition of your hair much better than others. Once again, it is possible to use both a permanent wave and a permanent coloring agent on the same hair, though not at the same sitting. But many well-known hairdressers caution against it—just too much of the natural shine and protective cuticle of the hair shaft is destroyed.

Chapter III:
Basic Facts about Skin

Skin is the largest organ of your body—it's everywhere. Of course, the skin that concerns us most is the skin that shows the most. And that means first of all, the face. After that we worry about our hands, feet, legs, and body skin. In youth, we fight acne. As we get older, acne tends to fade, only to be replaced by wrinkles, crow's feet, age spots, and general loss of tone. The three great enemies of perfect skin are hormones, aging, and light.

Hormones have a lot to do with acne because they control the production of sebum, or skin oil. A little sebum is what you need to keep the skin supple, smooth, bathed in its own natural moisturizer. But a lot causes blocked pores, pimples, blackheads, and other eruptions. At least that's what dermatologists think is going on. The real culprit is the male hormone, androgen. But women's bodies produce androgens, too, at various times more than at others. And it's not only or even mainly the oil that gets to the surface of the skin that causes your face to break out—it's the oil that's trapped beneath the surface, that can't get to the surface to be washed away.

As you get older, the action of your hormones seems to calm down—and that's good, up to a point. But one day you wake up and realize that the skin you used to scrub with alcohol pads (I know one girl who washed with scouring cleanser. Please, don't take that as a recommendation!) is suddenly getting tight and dry.

Worse yet, most of us find sometime along about the mid-thirties that we have what has been called "combination" skin: it's greasy down the middle and dry around the edges. Now your skin begins to wrinkle—around the mouth, around the eyes. There's only one word for what you have to do to retard this process. (Nothing can *stop* it, no matter what they say.) The word is moisturize. Ideally, you should start a regular program of oil treatment for your skin the minute your natural oils reach a non-acne causing balance. We're not always aware of that exact moment however, so let's say after twenty-five. There are lots of moisturizers, and they do different things, but the important basic to keep in mind is that skin without a protective coating of oil loses water, and it's water in the tissues that keeps skin plump, firm, and young-looking.

Finally, there's light. I'll bet that came as a bit of a surprise to some of you, but it's true. Sunlight, *any* sunlight ages the skin. And it's not just a matter of drying effects—it's something more, like the gradual fading of furniture under the steady beating of sun. As you know, that happens even through windows, so you don't have to be a sun-worshipping tan freak to suffer at least some of the aging effects of old Sol. Naturally, you can't avoid daylight just to keep your skin from aging. It would help, but life is to live, not just to take care of your face. It does suggest, though, doesn't it, that Scarlett O'Hara and her crowd were onto something when they insisted that they couldn't be seen outdoors without their sunbonnets. The more you expose your skin, and especially the delicate skin of your face to wind, weather, and especially sun, the faster it ages. I know, there's nothing makes you look healthier than a nice tan, and it's the fashion these days, as it wasn't in Scarlett's, to look like a little brown child just come from the beach. But have you ever seen how people who work (or play) in the sun all the time look when they're about forty-five? Not to mention sixty-five.

I know you've seen the syndrome—skin like leather, and badly kept leather at that. Looking like a grownup sun pixie today can guarantee you'll look like a tough old turkey tomorrow. Others have said it, and I know you're going to be hearing it more and more often as the evidence rolls in: stay out of the sun.

Extremely cold weather can damage your skin, too, particularly if you have fair skin, and a tendency toward broken capillaries. And it's well-known that too much alcohol can give you permanently ruddy cheeks and a big red nose of the kind that looks lots better on Rudolph than on you. If you ski, or if you live in a place where the winters are cold but you have to go out anyway, be sure your skin is extra well protected at these times. For ski trips, you need a sun block, plus moisturizers, and you need to re-apply them from time to time so the effects don't wear off. The same kind of protection—in moderation—is in order for trips to the store or walks with the kids in winter weather wherever you are. More and more people are jogging or cross-country skiing in the cities, no matter what the weather, and that's wonderful for our bodies, but rough on our faces. (Always wear gloves, on these outings, or you'll have to worry about old-looking, wrinkled *hands,* too.)

What to Do About Acne

To begin at the beginning, we'll talk about the chief problem confronting young skin—acne and its attendant over-production of oil. To tell you the truth right away, the real causes of acne are still at least somewhat shrouded in mystery. The latest thinking contradicts some of the truisms that the older ones of us were raised on. For instance, I, like many other girls my age, gave up chocolate for the duration. Not a bad idea, I suppose, if you want to maintain a good figure, but doctors now say it has nothing to do with causing or aggravating acne. When I think of all the Hershey bars I could have eaten when I was a perpetually skinny fourteen! But never mind. The facts are out now: Hard cheese, chocolate candy, nuts, fried chicken and all those good things won't make your face break out. Conversely, avoiding them won't keep your face from breaking out, so you might as well live a little before you have to start watching your weight.

There's such a thing as too much cleaning of troubled skin, something they would ever have believed around the halls of my high school. If you've just come up from a session in the mines or a few hours of gardening, of course you'll want to clean the surface dirt off your face. But scrubbing and scrubbing and scrubbing to remove every trace of natural oils (and a few layers of epidermis) can make your breakout blues worse, not better. Blackheads are not, repeat not, caused by having a dirty face. They're caused by that old villain sebum, trapped at the entrance to a pore and blocking further oil from escaping naturally to the surface of the skin. Gentle washing will help unblock the pores in time, but abrasive scrubbing will probably lead to infection and much more serious pimples.

Here's more bad news: if you think your acne will magically disappear when you hit eighteen or twenty-one, or when you get married, think again. (Having a baby can help, though, but usually only for the period of actual pregnancy.) Actually, hormone activity can cause occasional eruptions throughout life, even into old age. But usually these are restricted to once-in-a-while blemishes after the initial teen turbulence. Scarring, that hangover bane of the acne-prone, can happen at any age if you pick and squeeze. As many have found to their sorrow, acne scars persist long after the offending blemishes have disappeared.

Can anything be done about acne scars? Well, yes, but you wouldn't want to go through it unless your problem is really pretty severe. The chief methods of reducing pits and craters left by acne are both forms of abrasion, think sandpaper and you'll get the general idea. Real sandpaper isn't used, but what is used is quite harsh—either a chemical, in which case it's chemabrasion, or a really nasty-looking stainless steel brush that is rotated near the face, in which case it's dermabrasion. In either case, there is some pain, and an annoying period of healing when your face looks a lot like it has a bad case of poison ivy. So who needs it? I think you'll know who you are if you do. Obviously, if your difficulty is one little scar that keeps your chin from looking like a model's, I don't think you'll want to go through the expense and discomfort these treatments involve. On the other hand, if your life is really being blighted by a face that looks like a dormant volanco, you probably won't have to think two minutes to know that you can put up with a couple of weeks of itching and oozing face to get a smoother skin. My advice: if you're set on undergoing abrasive treatment, find the best dermatologist in the world, and get there if you can. The success of the process has a lot to do with the skill of the practitioner.

There are a few other treatments for acne scars, such as skin grafts and silicone injections, but there's also controversy over just how well these work and whether the risks are worth the improvement. For those with just a few scars that reason tells you aren't very important but subjective reflection tells you are just *odious,* a few tips. First of all, makeup can do wonders. One of the things a cover-up stick or good foundation can cover best is a scar of the idented type. And makeup stays put on scars better than on the rest of your face. Second, time fades scars: not completely, but substantially. Third, a light golden tan (not, ever, the leather-look darkness of the sun worshipper) can minimize scars. But watch out for the sun, as we've said before. It may turn out, after it's too late, that you would rather have gone through life with that scar on your chin showing than thousands of little wrinkles at the corners of your eyes.

Oily Skin

Everyone has oily skin, dry skin, or a combination of both. If there's anyone anywhere who has perfect skin at this moment—neither too wet nor too dry—you can be sure she won't have it next week. Models and actresses and natural beauties whose bone structure takes your breath away are all reduced to their common humanity by the universality of skin problems. Everyone needs drying agents (astringents) and moisturizers (face creams), and most of us need them both.

The best and easiest way to determine your skin type is to just think back on your experience with your skin (by which I mean mainly your face) over the years. If your forehead and nose and chin tend to get shiny and greasy as the day goes by, if you're troubled by blackheads in these areas, if you have large pores on nose, cheeks, and chin, you fit the usual pattern for oily skin. The clincher: do you *wake up* with oil in those aforementioned spots? That's what happens to people with oily skin. But it doesn't mean that you ought to wash constantly with harsh soap and avoid moisturizers.

The base of any skin-care program is a regular facial. That means different things to different skin types, and you'll have a chance to experiment to your heart's content during your 14-Day program. Generally, drying agents such as alcohol are only used directly on eruptions unless you're very young. This is true for those with oily or combination skin as well as for those with dry skin. Alcohol is just too harsh for over-thirty faces. For your oily skin, the program might be a deep-cleaning via steam (not really steam, that would scald you: just hot water vapor), a masque to lift out the cloggings in your pores, then moisturizing. But don't suppose that such treatment sessions are only for those with dry skin. They're essential to the looks and life of your face, too, they just have to be geared to your special needs.

Dry Skin

Here's how to tell if your skin is dry: Does the skin of your face get to feeling like it's a size too small for what it has to cover, especially in the winter? Does the wind and weather seem to be harder on your face than on others, actually peeling or flaking it sometimes? Have you been noticing little lines around the stress points—eyes and mouth—since before your mother let you have your first pair of high heels? That's what you've got, then, dry skin. In my opinion, and you know this is sincere because dry skin is not my problem, this is the skin type that produces that truly beautiful, porcelain skin that seems to be as without flaw as an orchid. Enlarged pores, you see, the bane of all of us with oily or in-between skin, don't afflict our dry-skinned sisters. But this is also the type of skin that ages the fastest if it's abused or just not given enough tender loving care. Be warned.

The regular facial is a must for dry-skinned women, too. But that's not all. An absolutely religious ritual of moisturizing should be started by such women as soon as teenage oil problems have settled down. And if you're a teenager who doesn't seem to have any pimples, blackheads or excess oil, be on your guard. It probably means you're going to have "laugh lines" when the rest of your friends are still spending most of their pocket money on Clearasil. Start moisturizing now, even if you don't think you need it. Take my word for it, five minutes night and morning with a jar of cream can save you many hours and dollars later on.

For women with all skin types, a moisturizer is only the start of a complete treatment program. But it's the essential. If you were scheduled to be exiled to a desert island and you could only take one cosmetic, forget the lipstick. For lasting beauty, there's only one reasonable choice, and that's your moisturizing cream.

When we get to your individual facial program, we'll discuss which skin products (given you live in a fair-sized town or near one and not on a desert island) you really ought to have for younger-longer skin, and which will only make your skin worse.

Professional Care

What's the single nicest thing you can do for your face on a one-shot basis? You know already, I'm sure: get yourself a professional facial. It's relaxing, good for the morale, and truly, though temporarily, beautifying. After you've finished an hour or two under the hands of a really competent skin-care expert in a salon, you'll feel babied, loved, rested, and lovely. And you'll look that way, too. How you feel about yourself and your life tends to show in your face, and a short time-out for a purely self-indulgent professional facial can have immediate positive results on your psyche as well as on your skin.

Depending on your resources, you may want to keep it up with regular monthly facial appointments, or you may want to duplicate the effects at home. Either way, every woman should have at least one salon facial. It's not quite as relaxing when you're the giver as well as the receiver, but you'll want to try to duplicate the relaxed and relaxing atmosphere of a good skin salon as well as the products and their use. How can you do it if you don't try it once?

While you're in the capable hands of the cosmetician, watch everything she does. (Don't fall asleep, however great the temptation. Someday, no matter how rich you are, you'll want to try this at home.) If you wonder about the purpose of a certain procedure, don't be shy about asking. And be suspicious of anyone who seems reluctant to tell. Either they don't know what they're about, or they have something to hide. Of course, you won't get salon professionals to tell the recipes of their masques and creams. Those are trade secrets, as jealously guarded and frantically spied upon as atomic arsenals. But as to what this cleansing solution or that pink goo is supposed to do for you, you have every right to know, and there's no reason why you shouldn't be told. Once you know, you can compare products to see which one you can use for the same effect. You can also give your facial a critical once-over to see if it produced the promised results.

I also recommend a professional makeup job, just once, although not necessarily on the same day as your facial, unless you have plenty of time, money, and patience at being manipulated. For most of us, an hour or two is pleasant, but after that it gets to be trying. (Think about that the next time you sigh for a model's life. They're poked, painted, and pounded practically from morning to night—not to mention pinned, sometimes, when the fitter gets overzealous.) You may not want to do your face just the way the expert does, but you'll pick up some priceless tips from watching him or her work. I think most professional makeup jobs tend to be on the heavy side for most ordinary lifestyles, at least for day wear. But most amateur jobs tend to be not enough or lopsided in their emphasis. If you consider your salon makeup session a lesson or tutorial session—which means, once again, that you'll have to pay attention— you'll consider it well worth the price. Another tip. If there's just no cash in the piggy bank for a salon makeup job, take your naked face—no makeup, please—down to the demonstration counters of your major local department store. You know the place I mean, it's usually on the first floor, and the whole area—counters and counters of beauty products and immaculate sales women with perfectly done faces—exudes a perfumy warmth. A nice place to take your face, anytime. Somewhere in that pink-and-gold maze will be someone who's doing faces to demonstrate her products. Or if she isn't, she will, on the suggestion that you want to buy. Sit down and let her show you all the tricks they showed her when the company gave her their sales training course. Try to pick a woman whose makeup job you like—ninety-nine times out of a hundred, she did it herself. Although the quality of instruction you'll get may rival that in any salon, you'll have to have your face done right out there in public, in front of everyone. But it's a much better deal than a beauty-school haircut, and cheaper, too. You don't have to buy a thing if you don't want to.

The Outdoor Life of the Skin

There was a time when women who had the leisure to do so cultivated a deathly pallor such as one only sees in hospitals and prisons today. Surprisingly, it turns out that it was better for the skin, and for the long life of the young look than our "healthy", outdoorsy way of life today. Of course, sitting indoors fanning yourself isn't very good for the tone and condition of the rest of you, and nobody in her right mind would advocate a return to the good old days when heavy exercise for a lady of quality was ringing for a servant to bring the tea. (It wasn't within the means of the servant, unfortunately, to sit around growing interestingly pale.)

In our time, working women and women who've never had to work spend a good part of their time in sports and other outdoor activity. This is not even to count the millions who actually lie on their backs with their faces turned up toward the sun, trying to get the healthy look via self-cooking. Since I don't approve of sun bathing as such, I'll talk about that last. But what about the unavoidable exposure to sun, wind, and water that an ordinary active lifestyle must entail? How can we keep from aging in the face just when we've finally learned how to keep our bodies young and alive?

Moisturizing, of course, is part of the answer. Wind, heat, cold, and water all dry the skin by evaporating or washing away the oils that lock our own natural moisture in. I'd say that every woman should moisturize morning and evening and after bathing. For women who also jog or play tennis or garden or whatever activity gets you out in the weather, there should be an extra moisturizing session before you go out. It's far better to protect your face from drying than to try to correct damage already done.

As for the sun, the only sensible course is a sunscreen lotion, applied winter or summer to every part of you that will have any lengthy exposure. A sunscreen, to be perfectly clear, is a cream or lotion that completely blocks the ultraviolet rays (the ones that tan, and burn, and age your skin) from reaching through to you. It is not the same thing as a suntan lotion, most of which are designed to screen out only some of the ultra-violet light so that your tan builds up slowly. True, this is better than sunburn, but even better is no exposure at all.

Why am I so down on sunshine? Don't those glorious rays make us all feel relaxed, warm, happy and exhilarated? I admit they do. But some pleasures simply must be foregone for the cause of reason and the long run. Don't we all look better with a bit of a tan—doesn't it even out our color, hide flaws and lines, make us look strong and young and full of the joy of living? True, again. And back in the days before I found out what damage the sun could do, I loved lying around the pool or the beach working on my tan, too. But there comes a time when the evidence against some practice or other gets too strong to ignore, and that's what's happened with sun. Not only has science found out that sunlight is the prime cause of aging, wrinkles, sagging, and just general destruction of the skin, but sun, especially sunburn, has been implicated as the chief cause of skin cancer. People who work outside in the sun have the highest incidence of skin cancer—unless they happen to be blacks or other dark-skinned people who have the natural protection of extra pigmentation.

Because that's what your skin is trying to do, you know, when it exhibits the reaction known as tanning. It's trying to build up a barrier against the sun with the body's pigment—melanin—so that further damage from direct light will be minimized. When you think of tanning that way—as a sort of callus of color formed by the skin in trying to shield itself from all that sun you're poring on, it doesn't seem quite so attractive, does it? If it seems that I'm trying to talk you out of your sunbathing habits, you're right. I know it's a hard pattern to break, particularly since the positive results—nice golden tan—show up right away, while the negative results are long-term, not appearing for years after the fact. But we in the last quarter of the twentieth century have had to learn to deal with many of the long-term consequences of our actions, just because our knowledge is expanding. For the first time, we are in a position to know and control many of the effects of what we do. It seems to me that the fashion for a tan skin began somewhere—some say with the return of Coco Chanel from a Mediterranean vacation—and it might just as well end with us.

But suppose you can't be convinced that zero sunbathing is the way to go. Suppose your doctor told you the sun was good for your acne or your psoriasis or your ego. Does that mean you have to resign yourself to looking like an old shoe in fifteen years so you can have your little bit of sunshine today? Not really. I say again, your skin will be at its best in those distant days if you use a sunscreen all the time and never get tan. (Look for the ingredient PABA or para-aminobenzoic acid on the label to tell if you've got hold of a true sunscreen). But if you must sun, at least proceed with caution. Sunburn—what happens when you take too much too soon—is incredibly bad for your skin. One single bad sunburn can lead to skin cancer—though it sometimes takes a long time to show up. So, if you insist on sunbathing, and this may seem like a paradox at first, plan to spend a lot of time in the sun.

The reason I say you should spend a lot of time getting

your tan is that you should limit your exposures to only a few minutes a day. It doesn't add up to a lot of hours, just a lot of days. Begin your tanning with a mere ten minutes. I mean literally ten. And be sure your brief period in the sun doesn't come between 10 a.m. and 2 p.m., which is the period of the day when the sun is highest in the sky and the path of its rays to you is most direct. Remember, even if you don't see blisters, redness, and swelling, you may be hurting your skin by pushing it too fast into the blessed condition of tan.

And don't forget your sunglasses or goggles, whether you get your exposure at sea level or on top of a mountain. First, there are all those nasty squint lines that you don't want to see staring back when you look in the mirror six months from now. Second, and even more important, the eyes aren't immune to damage by the sun. Tests have shown that there is a wide variation in the ability of various sunglasses on the market to filter out the burning and glaring rays. Don't choose a pair because they have the best-looking frames or polarized lenses, or the color that's in. Choose them because they seem to you to be the best at reducing squint and glare. You may have to step out of the store to really test this out—not possible at some of our more suspicious establishments. But take the time to get a good pair, even if you have to shop around a bit. Your eyes and your mirror will thank you.

Chapter IV:
Cosmetic Surgery

If Jacqueline Kennedy as First Lady ushered in the age of the bouffant hairdo and the pillbox hat, Betty Ford seems to have made this the age of the face-lift. Suddenly, it seems everyone is doing it, or at least telling about it. It used to be that when a gentleman or a lady decided to have those sagging eyelids lifted, the chin re-molded, the nose bobbed, they quietly "vacationed" in Mexico or some other suitably remote place until all traces of the after-effects had gone. Subsequently, they discreetly side-stepped inquiries about the suddenly younger face except to closest friends and Truman Capote. As Russell Baker has observed, wrinkles are as out as the Nehru jacket. (Characteristically, however, Baker isn't having a face job, just in case wrinkles should come back in and catch him unfashionably smooth.)

Most of us aren't in a position to have every little blemish and wrinkle stitched and snipped out of existence, but there are some times, even in the lives of us normal, well-adjusted non-movie stars, when it seems that that one glaring flaw, if it were only removed, would make such a difference in its absence. Or maybe your face used to be fine, but it's lately started to sag and bag in ways that make you say, "I'm too young to look that old." Fads aside, there are many legitimate reasons why you might want, at some time in your life, to investigate cosmetic surgery. Here, then, is my quick course in what it can, and cannot do.

The Nose

The "nose job" is still the most common operation for the average plastic surgeon. There are several reasons, I think, but the basic one has to be that from the point of view of the patient, the nose job is still the most successful kind of plastic surgery. For one thing, there are really no visible scars with this operation. No matter what you've heard, that's not true of a face lift, a tummy tightening, any other kind of self-improvement by surgery. Scars are often small and cleverly buried in folds of skin, but they're always there, and there's no way to tell for sure until after the surgery whether your scars will fade to insignificance or not. But in rhinoplasty, as the nose job is called in the trade, incisions are made *inside* the nose, so nothing ever shows. Another good reason is that rhinoplasty is a highly developed art. If you have a good surgeon, you'll get a good-looking nose.

Can you choose the nose you want from a big book of possible noses? Not quite. How your new nose turns out depends partly on the doctor, partly on the rest of your face, and partly on how your body heals. A standard joke in plastic surgery circles is the "signature" nose. This happens when a doctor seems to get stuck in a rut, producing face after face with the same nose. The best strategy when shopping for a plastic surgeon, particularly if it's rhinoplasty you want, is to personally interview several women who've had the same operation from the same doctor. Failing that, you can ask to look at photos of the doctor's past work. There's nothing wrong with the signature nose, by the way, if it happens to be right for your face. It's when it doesn't fit that it's bad.

The very best kind of nose job, because it has the highest success rate, is the kind where you just have the bump taken out of the middle. To do this, the surgeon breaks the bone, (ouch) removes excess material through the nostrils, then re-sets the bone in its new, straight pattern. Of course, you don't really feel all this, not while it's happening, because you've been numbed with a local anesthesia. But there is some discomfort associated with the post-operative period, and you'll be black and blue over extensive areas of your face, including your eyeballs. Most people choose to lie low for a week or two after a nose job. Less satisfying procedures involve re-shaping of the tip of the nose and the nostrils—trickier stuff, and it sometimes leaves visible scars. If you have a past history of slow or poor healing or lumpy scars, you're not a prime candidate for most plastic surgery.

The Face

After the nose, the second most common area to be corrected by cosmetic surgery is the little patch between the eyes and the eyebrows. This operation is just as popular with men as it is with women. As the face gets older, some people (and your genes determine how prone you are to this) develop such a heavy fold above the eyes that the skin comes down and rests on the eye lashes. The not-quite-candid say they had their eyelid surgery because the fold was obscuring vision. Most of the time, though, the real reason is because all that skin piled up on top of the eye makes the eyes look smaller and the whole face look squinty and old.

The "eye-lift" procedure has a fairly good chance of leaving a virtually unnoticeable scar, because the incision is hidden in the place where the open eye folds back. Whoever you sleep with might see the scars, but they'll be invisible when you're awake. But, unlike the nose job, eyework really can't be done over and over until you're satisfied. If your surgeon gets it wrong the first time, you may end up with pulled-down eyes that look as though your face were too tight around them. Some of the less adept have been known to produce eyes that literally won't close, an even more serious consequence than botched appearance. As with every other surgical procedure, there is always a slight risk of complications—from the anesthesia, from the shock to the body, from accidental severing of what shouldn't have been severed. It's always important around the eyes to be ultra-careful.

Besides having a tuck taken in your upper lids, you can have bags removed from below the eyes, or have your eyebrows and sometimes the whole forehead lifted. The eyebrow-lift makes the most prominent scar of all these operations, and unless you want to have to wear eyebrow pencil all the time to cover it, you'll be disappointed in the results. Although we seem to be much freer in admitting that we've had cosmetic surgery these days, most of us still haven't reached the frame of mind where we think the scars are attractive symbols of status. Always remember that all surgery leaves scars, and all but rhinoplasty leave them on the outside, where they can be seen. Yes, doctors try to keep them tiny and hide them in folds or in the hairline, but a lot depends on how well you heal and whether or not you tend to scar easily and permanently. You can't even take a tuck in a dress without having the line show—how much less in a face?

Chin

The real "face-lift" involves tightening up the lower third of the face by pulling up the skin at the hairline. You can get the same effect temporarily by wearing a specially-designed wig that pulls your face tight as it covers your hair. The so-called "mini-lift" is, rather disappointingly, not a little bit of a chin-lift, but the same kind of procedure on the upper third of the face—it's good if you have an unusual amount of forehead-wrinkling, but won't do anything for the effects of gravity on that all-important jaw and neck area. What this operation is best for is that sagging, jowly look that identifies you as someone whose face has been experiencing the effects of planetary attraction for a good long time. What it isn't good for is thousands of tiny laugh lines around the mouth (or eyes) or for those two deep, curving lines that indicate just where and how you always smile. (Smiling, by the way, is a wonderful instant cosmetic for the aging face. We tend to forget, as we get older, that our faces in total relaxation look more and more solemn, even angry, just because they are sagging ever-so-slightly downward. If you cultivate a slight smile, you'll look less forbidding.) P.S. Just as nobody may have told you before about the black-and-blue eyeballs associated with the nose job, be warned here that your face may look unnaturally tight—and feel that way, too—for a while after a face-lift. Any time after cosmetic surgery is a good time to schedule that solitary vacation in Brazil or Zen retreat you've been contemplating. It's never like those old movies where the heroine takes off the bandages and finds she's a dead ringer for Olivia DeHaviland. Unless you're prepared, you may think they've turned you into the Bride of Frankenstein instead.

Ears

If you're a good bet for ear-surgery (otoplasty), you'll know it. This isn't for people whose ears stick out so slightly that they're the only ones who've ever noticed it. Even if your ears stand out more than that, it's only important if you mind. But if your greatest hope is that nobody will call you Dumbo when you walk into a strange room perhaps this is the operation for you. If your ears do stick out quite a lot, it means you have extra material behind them to be removed. That's pretty much what happens during the procedure. Since the scars are behind your ears, where nobody but your mother has ever been known to look, they're usually almost as good as invisible.

Body

Until maybe twenty years ago, nobody but strippers and movie stars had cosmetic surgery anyplace but the face. That's because most of us don't reveal our bodies much, and were content to camouflage the effects of aging and gravity with support garments and substantial fabrics that hid the sags. But the string bikini and the T-shirt have changed all that for good. Exercise and diet can do a lot to keep you looking young and trim below the neck, but they can't do it all. The breasts, for example, while supported to some degree by muscles, contain no muscle themselves, and consequently can't be exercised back into their teen firmness and height, no matter how many hours a day you spend at the gym. Often, too, a stretched and sagging abdomen or bulges at the tops of the thighs prove intractable, even if you're more than rigorous about your diet and exercise. (And some of us, of course, would prefer surgery to rigor, anytime.)

I think I'm safe in saying that body-sculpting operations are slightly more controversial and perhaps slightly less satisfactory to the owners of the bodies than cosmetic surgery on the face. For one thing, these operations are newer, and there is still considerable difference of opinion within the medical profession about the best way to go about things. Some surgeons, for instance, swear by gel implants in the breast-augmenting procedure, while others use only the saline-solution implant. In either case, the substance is enclosed in a sac or envelope—most often made of silicone—so that none of the fluid or gel can leak away from the site and get into the circulation. But both doctors and patients disagree as to which type of implant leaves the breast feeling (to you and to others) the most natural. Both types of augmentation seem to look pretty good, by the way, but looks aren't all we care about. We want the breasts to feel like real breasts when we touch them, and we want them to have the same capacity for sensation they had before.

In a certain percentage of the cases, it doesn't work out like that. Whether the factors involved in breast sensitivity are entirely physical or partly psychological isn't known, but there have been disappointed women (and men), so stand advised.

Breasts can also be reduced in size and/or lifted. All of these operations leave scars in visible places, though those made by highly competent hands seem to fade to the point where only a doctor would notice. If you're married to a doctor, don't try to hide anything from him. In breast-reduction, the nipple often has to be moved upward, too, so that it will still be the center of attention. That means more scars, a longer procedure, and generally a bit more discomfort. You should also know that some doctors feel that any tampering with the tissues slightly increases the chance that something will go wrong with them later, including cancer. Other doctors don't go along with this, so trust the opinion of your regular medical advisor.

How about the rest of your body? Can you have plastic surgery on the stretch marks left over from your pregnancy or your big weight loss binge? Can you have your hips, thighs, bottom and stomach re-done? Of course. You may have read about Brazil's Dr. Ivo Pitanguy, who specializes in carving up the wealthy women of Rio so that they can fit into the teeny bikini of their choice. These operations inevitably leave long and sometimes lumpy scars, but the high-society women who patronize Dr. Pitanguy don't mind. One of his scars is something like a designers's signature on your shirt, if you like that sort of thing. Personally, though I don't mind having certain famous initials on my handbag or my suit, I'd balk at having them carved right in my side. Since my livelihood is based in a business that teaches women how to get their bodies in shape the natural way, I'm naturally partial to exercise in the right places rather than having yourself "sculpted." Besides, surgery is risky for your body and deals with appearance only, while exercise is good for the inner you—your heart, lungs, blood circulation—rather than just the part everyone can see. After all, you want to be around a long time to enjoy your new beauty, don't you?

Actually, the list of possible cosmetic procedures goes on and on. You can have the fine lines around your mouth sanded down via dermabrasion or chemabrasion (you'll remember those from the section on acne treatment. There is some pain and a rather long healing period, so the procedures aren't to be undertaken lightly.) You can have your abdominal skin adjusted so the stretch marks don't show, although you can't get rid of them completely. You can have your navel re-shaped (to fit the emerald given you by the Sheik, no doubt), or even have the deep lines of your mouth and forehead filled in with silicone. The chin can be augmented or reduced, and there's a surgical procedure for removing broken capillaries on the face or varicose veins on the legs.

The only place to get competent advice about whether or not any of these operations is right for you is from a really first-rate surgeon. Try to find one whose sub-specialty is the exact operation that you're interested in. A good doctor will not only be skilled in the surgery in question, but he or she will be able to judge whether the extent of your problem justifies the slight but very real risks plus the discomfort involved. Some people have cosmetic surgery out of boredom or because they're pathologically obsessed with having the perfect nose or breasts or whatever. Such patients will find a doctor somewhere to do their bidding—they just won't take no for an answer. But you should be willing to be talked out of cosmetic surgery if the best doctors agree you don't need it. After all, it's expensive, it's no fun under the best circumstances, and if your problem is slight to begin with, it won't make that much difference in your appearance. A prominent surgeon said to me that he was willing to do noses and ears and chins for psychological reasons, even if objective observers agreed that the patient didn't look so bad the way she was. "Anything else," he concluded, "and the drawbacks outweigh the benefits when it's purely a question of state-of-mind." Something to keep in mind when you examine your reasons for wanting plastic surgery.

Chapter V:
Basic Facts About
Physical Fitness

What it is.
In a technical sense, physical fitness can be viewed as a measure of the body's strength, stamina and flexibility. In more meaningful personal terms, it is a reflection of your ability to work with vigor and pleasure, without undue fatigue, with energy left for enjoying hobbies and recreational activities, and for meeting unforeseen emergencies. It relates to how you look and how you feel—and, because the body is not a compartment separate from the mind, it relates to how you feel mentally as well as physically.

Physical fitness is many-faceted. Basic to it are proper nutrition, adequate rest and relaxation, good health practices, and good medical and dental care.

But these are not enough. An essential element is physical activity—exercise for a body that needs it.

Why exercise?
Wherever there is muscle there is need of movement.

The human body contains more than 600 muscles;

overall, it is more than half muscle.

Muscles make possible every overt motion. They also push food along the digestive tract, suck air into the lungs, tighten blood vessels to raise blood pressure when you need more pressure to meet an emergency. The heart itself is a muscular pump.

Technological advances have changed our way of living, have made strenuous physical exertion largely unnecessary. The word "chore" has virtually gone out of use.
But the needs of the human body have not changed. Muscles are meant to be used. When they are not used, or not used enough, they deteriorate. If we are habitually inactive—if we succumb to the philosophy of easy living—we must then pay the price in decreased efficiency.

Research support for regular physical activity as an essential for healthful and vigorous living is increased constantly.

That we are, to a great degree, what our muscles make us—weak or strong, vigorous or lethargic—is a growing conviction among medical men.

Offering strong support for this conviction is the following observation by a former president of the American Medical Association: "It begins to appear that exercise is the master conditioner for the healthy and the major therapy for the ill."

A recent survey of a cross section of physicians—nearly 4,000—showed that almost all now believe strongly that positive health benefits, both physical and mental, accompany physical fitness resulting from regular, moderate exercise. It also revealed that the great majority have come to favor the inclusion of tests of physical fitness in periodic health examinations—and are convinced that physical fitness programs, which have been largely aimed at children, are even more necessary for adults.

Some specific benefits.
An obvious effect of regular exercise is the firming of flabby muscles.

In addition, research indicates that exercise produces beneficial changes in the functioning of internal organs—especially the heart, lungs and circulatory system. The heart beat becomes stronger and steadier, breathing becomes deeper and circulation improves.

Research lists these benefits experienced by people who, after a prolonged period of sedentary living, undertake a systematic conditioning program:
    Increased strength, endurance and coordination
    Increased joint flexibility
    Reduction of minor aches, pains, stiffness and soreness
    Correction of remediable postural defects
    Improvement in general appearance
    Increased efficiency with reduced expenditure of energy in performing both physical and mental tasks.
    Improved ability to relax and to voluntarily reduce tension
    Reduction of chronic fatigue

Exercise and chronic fatigue
Ranking today as one of the most frequently voiced of all complaints, chronic tiredness can stem from illness. But in many people, investigators report, it is the result of gradual deterioration of the body from lack of enough

vigorous physical activity.

Continual inactivity produces muscular atrophy and the individual soon becomes under-muscled for his weight. The result: he lacks the strength and endurance to do his daily work easily and efficiently.

One important end result of the increased muscular strength and general endurance provided by exercise is an increase in the body's capacity for carrying on normal daily activities, a pushing back of fatigue limits.

Valid research indicates that a fit person uses less energy for any given movement or effort than a flabby or weak person.

Exercise and the heart
An old-fashioned idea—that exercise may be bad for the heart—has been shown to be without scientific foundation. Not only that—it has been proven that appropriate exercise strengthens the heart.

A noted heart specialist recently commented: "The best insurance against coronary (heart) disease is exercise—lots of it."

Backing up this conviction is a growing body of evidence. It includes findings of lower cholesterol values in active people, faster clearing of fats from the blood after meals—and sharply reduced heart attack rates.

A recent study covering 120,000 American railroad employees revealed the heart attack incidence among sedentary office workers to be almost twice that of people working in the yards. Other studies—in the United States, England and elsewhere—also show a higher rate of heart attacks among the sedentary than among the physically active.

Additionally, the studies indicate that, when a heart attack does occur, the physically active person is more likely to recover. One possible reason: there is evidence that exercise may promote development of supplementary blood vessels which can take over the burden of nourishing the heart muscle when a coronary artery is blocked in a heart attack.

Exercise and aging
There is strong authoritative support for the concept that regular exercise can help prevent degenerative disease and slow down the physical deterioration that accompanies aging.

The evidence is conclusive: individuals who consistently engage in proper physical activity have better job performance records, fewer degenerative diseases, and probably a longer life expectancy that the population at large. By delaying the aging process, proper exercise also prolongs your active years.

A special note about weight
A common misconception is that exercise does not aid in weight control. This is not the case. Research shows:
   That fat piles up in most people by only a few calories a day;
   That an excess of only 100 calories a day can produce a 10-pound gain in a year—and that the extra calories could be burned up by a 15- to 20-minute daily walk;
   That obese people almost invariably tend to be much less active than those of normal weight;
   That individual weight, moreover, is a factor in energy expenditure. If you are overweight, you will burn up more calories in performing exercise than a person of normal weight.

According to studies by the Harvard School of Public Health, one-half hour of proper exercise each day can keep off or take off as much as 26 pounds a year.

Inactivity is the most important factor explaining the frequency of "creeping" overweight in modern Western society. And the consensus now among medical and health authorities is that the most effective way to take off weight and keep it off is through a program which combines proper exercise and reasonable diet.

If you need to lose weight, do so under the direction of your physician. Don't lose more than two pounds per week without his knowledge and consent. Determine to reduce gradually and consistently. Determine to develop proper eating habits. A change in diet—perhaps a change as slight as taking a little less sugar or none in beverages—may be all that is necessary to bring your weight down, especially if coupled with the essential exercise regime.

If you're handicapped
Where there is impairment or illness, any and all exercise should be medically prescribed and regulated.

Today, physicians are using exercise as an aid in combatting many chronic problems, including arthritis, asthma, diabetes and emphysema.

A common type of low back pain has been traced to weakened back muscles, and exercise has been used both to produce relief and to help prevent recurrences.

If you have a handicap, your doctor may find that some or many of the exercises given in this manual—perhaps with modifications—could be of value to you.

The Program For Women

Your complete basic program for achieving physical fitness with clear instructions and charts, progress records...everything you need.

Before you begin
A medical examination at least once a year is generally advisable for every adult. It's an excellent idea to get such an examination now before beginning your conditioning program.

Very probably your physician will be able to recommend that you proceed without restriction. If he should find any physical problems, he can take steps to correct it—and may have suggestions for modifying the program to make it more suitable for you.

Once you have had an examination, you can proceed confidently.

A reassuring word about muscles
As you make use of the program in the following pages, you need have no fear of becoming heavily, unattractively muscled. On the contrary:

With disuse or little use, muscles tend to become less elastic, weaker, softer. They lose tone.

The exercises you will be working with are designed to

firm your muscles, restore their tone, increase their strength and flexibility. Your appearance will improve as certain muscles—in the abdomen and back, for example—become more responsive, every move you make is likely to be easier and more graceful.

About the program

It assumes that you have not been engaging recently in consistent, vigorous, all-around physical activity—even though, in housework or other daily routines, you have put some muscles to extensive use.

It starts with an orientation or "get-set" series of exercises that will allow you to bring all major muscles into use easily and painlessly.

There are then five graded levels.

As you move from one to the next, you will be building toward a practical and satisfying level of fitness.

By building gradually, progressively, you will be building soundly.

What the exercises are for

There are three general types—warmup exercises, conditioning exercises and circulatory activities.

The warmup exercises stretch and limber up the muscles and speed up the action of the heart and lungs, thus preparing the body for greater exertion and reducing the possibility of unnecessary strain.

The conditioning exercises are systematically planned to tone up abdominal, back, leg, arm and other major muscles.

The circulatory activities produce contractions of large muscle groups for relatively longer periods than the conditioning exercises—to stimulate and strengthen the circulatory and respiratory systems.

The plan calls for doing 10 mild exercises during the orientation period and, thereafter, the warmup exercises and the seven conditioning exercises listed for each level. The first six exercises of the orientation program are used as warmup exercises throughout the graded levels.

When it comes to the circulatory activities, you choose one each workout. Alternately running and walking, skipping rope, running in place—all are effective. You can choose running and walking on a pleasant day, one of the others for use indoors when the weather is inclement. You can switch about for variety.

How you progress
A sound physical conditioning program should take into account your individual tolerance—your ability to execute a series of activities without undue discomfort or fatigue. It should provide for developing your tolerance by increasing the work load so you gradually become able to achieve more and more with less and less fatigue and with increasingly rapid recovery.

As you move from level to level, some exercises will be modified so they call for increased effort.

Others will remain the same but you will build more strength and stamina by increasing the number of repetitions.

You will be increasing your fitness another way as well.

At level 1, your objective will be to gradually reduce,

from workout to workout, the "breathing spells" between exercises until you can do the seven conditioning exercises without resting. You will proceed in the same fashion with the more difficult exercises and increased repetitions at succeeding levels. You will find the program designed—the progression carefully planned—to make this feasible. You will be able to proceed at your own pace, competing with yourself rather than with anyone else—and this is of great importance for sound conditioning.

Note: Gradually speeding up, from workout to workout, the rate at which you do each exercise will provide greater stimulation for the circulatory and respiratory systems and also help to keep your workouts short. However, the seven conditioning exercises should not be a race against time. Perform each exercise correctly to insure maximum benefit.

Choosing your goal
There is no need to pick the level to which you want to go—now.

Many women will be able to advance through the first three levels. While the fourth is challenging, some women will be able to achieve it. The fifth is one which only extremely vigorous, well-conditioned women will reach.

The level of fitness you can reach depends upon your age, your body's built-in potential capacity and previous conditioning. It also depends upon your state of mind; as you know, when you want to do something and believe you can, it is much easier to do than otherwise.

While there will be no dramatic overnight changes, gradually over the next weeks and months, as you progress through the first levels, you will begin to notice a new spring in your step, a new ease with which you accomplish your ordinary daily activities. You will find yourself with more energy left at the end of the working day and a new zest for recreation in the evening. Quite likely, you will be sleeping more soundly than you have slept for many years and waking more refreshed in the morning.

After completing the early levels, you may come to realize that you can—and want to—go further. Go as far as you can.

The important point is that, no matter what level you choose, you will greatly improve your physical fitness and you will be able to maintain the improvement and continue to enjoy the benefits.

When and how often to work out
To be most beautiful, exercise should become part of your daily routine—as much so as bathing and dressing.

Five workouts a week are called for throughout the program.

You can choose any time that's convenient. Preferably, it should be the same time every day—but it doesn't matter whether it's upon arising, at some point during the morning or afternoon, or in the evening.

How long at each level
Your objective at each level will be to reach the point where you can do all the exercises called for, for the number of times indicated, without resting between exercises.

But, start slowly.

It cannot be emphasized enough that by moving forward gradually you will be moving forward solidly, avoiding sudden strains and excesses that could make you ache and hold you back for several days.

If you find yourself at first unable to complete any exercises—to do continuously all the repetitions called for—stop when you encounter difficulty. Rest briefly, then take up where you left off and complete the count. If you have difficulty at first, there will be less and less with succeeding workouts.

Stay at each level for at least three weeks. If you have not passed the prove-out test at the end of that time, continue at the same level until you do. The prove-out test calls for performing—in three consecutive workouts—the seven conditioning exercises without resting and satisfactorily fulfilling the requirements for one circulatory activity.

A measure of your progress
You will, of course, be able to observe the increase in your strength and stamina from week to week in many ways— including the increasing facility with which you do the exercises at a given level.

In addition, there is a 2-minute step test you can use to measure and keep a running record of the improvement in your circulatory efficiency, one of the most important of all aspects of fitness.

The immediate response of the cardiovascular system to exercise differs markedly between well-conditioned individuals and others. The test measures the response in terms of pulse rate taken shortly after a series of steps up and down onto a bench or chair.

Although it does not take long, it is necessarily vigorous. Stop if you become overly fatigued while taking it. You should not try it until you have completed the orientation period.

The test

Use any sturdy bench or chair 15-17 inches in height.

    Count 1—Place right foot on bench.

    Count 2—Bring left foot alongside of right and stand erect.

    Count 3—Lower right foot to floor.

    Count 4—Lower left foot to floor.

    REPEAT the 4-count movement 30 times a minute for two minutes.

    THEN sit down on bench or chair for two minutes.

    FOLLOWING the 2-minute rest, take your pulse for 30 seconds.

    Double the count to get the per-minute rate. (You can find the pulse by applying middle and index finger of one hand firmly to the inside of the wrist of the other hand, on the thumb side.)

Record your score for future comparisons. In succeeding tests—about once every two weeks—you probably will find your pulse rate becoming lower as your physical condition improves.

Three important points:

    1. For best results, do not engage in physical activity for at least 10 minutes before taking the test. Take it at about the same time of day and always use the same bench or chair.

    2. Remember that pulse rates vary among individuals. This is an individual test. What is important is not a comparison of your pulse rate with that of anybody else—but rather a record of how your own rate is reduced as your fitness increases.

    3. As you progress, the rate at which your pulse is lowered should gradually level off. This is an indication that you are approaching peak fitness.

Charts are provided for the orientation program and for

each of the five levels.

They list the exercises to be done and the goal for each exercise in terms of number of repetitions, distance, etc.

They also provide space in which to record your progress—(1) in completing the recommended 15 workouts at each level (2) in accomplishing the three prove-out workouts before moving on to a succeeding level, and (3) in the results as you take the step test from time to time.

A sample chart and progress record for one of the five levels is shown below.

You do the warmup exercises and the conditioning exercises along with one circulatory activity for each workout.

Check off each workout as you complete it. The last three numbers are for the prove-out workouts, in which the seven conditioning exercises should be done without resting. Check them off as you accomplish them.

You are now ready to proceed to the next level.

As you take the step test—at about 2-week intervals—enter your pulse rate from the preceding level. Enter it in the margin to the left of the new progress record and circle it so it will be convenient for continuing reference.

SAMPLE	GOAL

Warmup Exercises   Exercises 1-6 of Orientation program

Conditioning Exercises	Uninterrupted repetitions

1. Bend and stretch 10
2. Sprinter 6
3. Sitting stretch 15
4. Knee pushup................................12
5. Situp (fingers laced) 10
6. Leg raiser .... 10 each leg
7. Flutter kick 30

Circulatory activity (choose one each workout)

Jog-walk (jog 50, walk 50) ....½ mile
Rope (skip 30 secs.; rest 60 secs.)........... 3 series
Run in place (run 100, hop 25 - 2 cycles) .... 3 minutes

Water activities—See recommendations on page 106.

Your progress record 1 2 3 4 5 6 7 8 9 10 11 12 13 14 15
prove-out
workouts

Step test (pulse)

With the series of mild exercises listed in the chart and described on the following pages, you can get yourself ready—without severe aches or pains—for the progressive conditioning program.

Plan to spend a minimum of one week for preliminary conditioning. Don't hestiate to spend two weeks or three if necessary for you to limber up enough to accomplish all the exercises easily and without undue fatigue.

1. BEND & STRETCH

Starting position: Stand erect, feet shoulder-width

apart.

Action: Count 1. Bend trunk forward and down, flexing knees. Stretch gently in attempt to touch fingers to toes or floor. Count 2. Return to starting position.

Note: Do slowly, stretch and relax at intervals rather than in rhythm.

2. KNEE LIFT

Starting position: Stand erect, feet together, arms at sides.

Action: Count 1. Raise left knee as high as possible, grasping leg with hands and pulling knee against body while keeping straight. Count 2. Lower to starting position. Counts 3 and 4. Repeat with right knee.

3. WING STRETCHER

Starting position: Stand erect, elbows at shoulder height, fists clenched in front of chest.

Action: Count 1. Thrust elbows backward vigorously without arching back. Keep head erect, elbows at shoulder height. Count 2. Return to starting position.

4. HALF KNEE BEND

Starting position: Stand erect, hands on hips.

Action: Count 1. Bend knees halfway while extending arms forward, palms down. Count 2. Return to starting position.

Conditioning Exercises	Repetitions
*1. Bend and stretch	10
*2. Knee lift	10 left 10 right
*3. Wing stretcher	20
*4. Half knee bend	10
*5. Arm circles	15 each way
*6. Body bender	10 left 10 right
7. Prone arch	10
8. Knee pushup	6
9. Head and shoulder curl	5
10. Ankle stretch	15

Circulatory activity (choose one each workout)
Walking .... ½ mile
Rope (skip 15 secs.; rest 60 secs.)............ 3 series

* The first six exercises of the Orientation program will be used as warmup exercises throughout the graded levels. Step Test Record—After completing the orientation program, take the 2-minute step test. Record your pulse rate here: _____
This will be the base rate with which you can make comparisons in the future.

5. ARM CIRCLES

Starting position: Stand erect, arms extended sideward at shoulder height, palms up.

Action: Describe small circles backward with hands. Keep head erect. Do 15 backward circles. Reverse, turn palms down and do 15 small circles forward.

6. BODY BENDER

Starting position: Stand, feet shoulder-width apart, hands

behind neck, fingers interlaced.

Action: Count 1. Bend trunk sideward to left as far as possible, keeping hands behind neck. Count 2. Return to starting position. Counts 3 and 4. Repeat to the right.

7. PRONE ARCH

Starting position: Lie face down, hands tucked under thighs.
Action: Count 1. Raise head, shoulders, and legs from floor. Count 2. Return to starting position.

8. KNEE PUSHUP

Starting position: Lie on floor, face down, legs together, knees bent with feet raised off floor, hands on floor under shoulders, palms down.

Action: Count 1. Push upper body off floor until arms are fully extended and body is in straight line from head to knees. Count 2. Return to starting position.

9. HEAD AND SHOULDER CURL

Starting position: Lie on back, hands tucked under small of back, palms down.

Action: Count 1. Tighten abdominal muscles, lift head and pull shoulders and elbows off floor. Hold for four seconds. Count 2. Return to starting position.

10. ANKLE STRETCH

Starting position: Stand on a stair, large book, or block of wood, with weight on balls of feet and heels raised.
Action: Count 1. Lower heels. Count 2. Raise heels.

CIRCULATORY ACTIVITIES

WALKING: Step off at a lively pace, swing arms and breathe deeply.
ROPE: Any form of skipping or jumping is acceptable.

Gradually increase the tempo as your skill and condition improve.

1. TOE TOUCH

Starting Position: Stand at attention.

Action: Count 1. Bend trunk forward and down, keeping knees straight, touching fingers to ankles. Count 2. Bounce and touch fingers to top of feet. Count 3. Bounce and touch fingers to toes. Count 4. Return to starting position.

2. SPRINTER

Starting Position: Squat, hands on floor, fingers pointed forward, left leg fully extended to rear.

Action: Count 1. Reverse position of feet in bouncing movement, bringing left foot to hands, extending right leg backward—all in one motion. Count 2. Reverse feet again, returning to starting position.

3. SITTING STRETCH

Starting position: Sit, legs spread apart, hands on knees.

Action: Count 1. Bend forward at waist, extending arms as far forward as possible. Count 2. Return to starting position.

4. KNEE PUSHUP

Starting position: Lie on floor, face down, legs together, knees bent with feet raised off floor, hands on floor under shoulders, palms down.

Action: Count 1. Push upper body off floor until arms are fully extended and body is in straight line from head to knees. Count 2. Return to starting position.

5. SITUP (ARMS EXTENDED)

Starting position: Lie on back, legs straight and together, arms extended beyond head.

Action: Count 1. Bring arms forward over head, roll up to sitting position, sliding hands along legs, grasping ankles. Count 2. Roll back to starting position.

6. LEG RAISER

Starting position: Right side of body on floor, head resting on right arm.

Action: Lift left leg about 24″ off floor, then lower it. Do required number of repetitions. Repeat on other side.

WOMEN: LEVEL ONE   GOAL

Warmup Exercises	Exercises 1-6 of Orientation program

Conditioning Exercises	Uninterrupted repetitions
1. Toe touch	5
2. Sprinter	8
3. Sitting stretch	10
4. Knee pushup	8
5. Situp (arms extended)	5
6. Leg raiser	5 each leg
7. Flutter kick	20

Circulatory activity (choose one each workout)

Walking (120 steps a minute) ....½ mile
Rope (skip 30 secs.; rest 60 secs.)........... 2 series
Run in place (run 50; straddle hop 10 - 2 cycles).. 2 minutes

Water Activities—See recommendations on page 106.

See recommendations on page 106.

Your progress record 1 2 3 4 5 6 7 8 9 10 11 12 13 14 15
Prove-out
workouts

Step test (pulse)

7. FLUTTER KICK

Starting position: Lie face down, hands tucked under thighs.

Action: Arch the back, bringing chest and head up, then flutter kick continuously, moving the legs 8″ - 10″ apart. Kick from hips with knees slightly bent. Count each kick as one.

CIRCULATORY ACTIVITIES

WALKING—Maintain a pace of 120 steps per minute for a distance of ½ mile. Swing arms and breathe deeply.

ROPE—Skip or jump rope continuously using any form for 30 seconds and then rest 60 seconds. Repeat 2 times.

RUN IN PLACE—Raise each foot at least 4″ off the floor and jog in place. Count 1 each time left foot touches floor. Complete number of running steps called for in chart, then do specified number of straddle hops. Complete 2 cycles of alternate running and hopping for time specified on chart.

STRADDLE HOP—Starting position: At attention.

Action: Count 1. Swing arms sideward and upward, touching hands above head (arms straight) while simultaneously moving feet sideward and apart in a single jumping motion. Count 2. Spring back to starting position. Two counts in one hop.

1. TOE TOUCH

Starting position: Stand at attention.
Action: Count 1. Bend trunk forward and down, keeping knees straight, touching fingers to ankles. Count 2. Bounce and touch fingers to top of feet. Count 3. Bounce and touch fingers to toes. Count 4. Return to starting position.

2. SPRINTER

Starting position: Squat, hands on floor, fingers pointed forward, left leg fully extended to rear.

Action: Count 1. Reverse position of feet in bouncing movement, bringing left foot to hands, extending right leg backward—all in one motion. Count 2. Reverse feet again, returning to starting position.

3 SITTING STRETCH

Starting position: Sit, legs spread apart, hands on knees.
Action: Count 1. Bend forward at waist, extending arms as far forward as possible. Count 2. Return to starting position.

4. KNEE PUSHUP

Starting position: Lie on floor, face down, legs together, knees bent with feet raised off floor, hands on floor under shoulders, palms down.

Action: Count 1. Push upper body off floor until arms are full extended and body is in straight line from head to knees. Count 2. Return to starting position.

5. SITUP (FINGERS LACED)

Starting position: Lie on back, legs straight and feet spread approximately 1' apart. Fingers laced behind neck.

Action: Count 1. Curl up to sitting position and turn trunk to left. Touch right elbow to left knee. Count 2. Return to starting position. Count 3. Curl up to sitting position and turn trunk to right. Touch left elbow to right knee. Count 4. Return to starting position. Score one situp each time you return to starting position. Knees may be bent as necessary.

6. LEG RAISER

Starting position: Right side of body on floor, head resting on right arm.

Action: Lift left leg about 24″ off floor, then lower it. Do required number of repetitions. Repeat on other side.

WOMEN: LEVEL TWO

Warmup Exercises	Exercises 1-6 of Orientation Program

Conditioning Exercises	Uninterrupted repetitions
1. Toe touch	10
2. Sprinter	12
3. Sitting stretch	15
4. Knee pushup	12
5. Situp (fingers laced)	10
6. Leg raiser	10 each leg
7. Flutter kick	30

Circulatory activity (choose one each workout)

Jog-walk (jog 50, walk 50) .... ½ mile
Rope (skip 30 secs.; rest 60 secs.)............ 3 series
Run in place (run 80, hop 15-2 cycles ...... 3 minutes

Water Activities—see recommendations on page 106.

Your Progress Record 1 2 3 4 5 6 7 8 9 10 11 12 13 14 15
Prove-out
workouts

Step test (pulse)

7. FLUTTER KICK

Starting position: Lie face down, hands tucked under thighs.

Action: Arch the back, bringing chest and head up, then flutter kick continuously, moving the legs 8"-10" apart. Kick from hips with knees slightly bent. Count each kick as one.

CIRCULATORY ACTIVITIES

JOG-WALK—Jog and walk alternately for number of paces indicated on chart for distance specified.
ROPE—Skip or jump rope continuously using any form for 30 seconds and then rest 60 seconds. Repeat 3 times.
RUN IN PLACE—Raise each foot at least 4" off floor and jog in place. Count 1 each time left foot touches floor. Complete number of running steps called for in chart,

then do specified number of straddle hops. Complete 2 cycles of alternate running and hopping for time specified on chart.

STRADDLE HOP—Starting position: At attention.

Action: Count 1. Swing arms sideward and upward, touching hands above head (arms straight) while simultaneously moving feet sideward and apart in a single jumping motion. Count 2. Spring back to starting position. Two counts in one hop.

1. TOE TOUCH

Starting position: Stand at attention

Action: Count 1. Bend trunk forward and down, keeping knees straight, touching fingers to ankles. Count 2. Bounce and touch fingers to top of feet. Count 3. Bounce and touch fingers to toes. Count 4. Return to starting position.

2. SPRINTER

Starting position: Squat, hands on floor, fingers pointed forward, left leg fully extended to rear.

Action: Count 1. Reverse position of feet in bouncing movement, bringing left foot to hands, extending right leg backward—all in one motion. Count 2. Reverse feet again, returning to starting position.

3. SITTING STRETCH (FINGERS LACED)

Starting position: Sit, legs spread apart, fingers laced behind neck.

Action: Count 1. Bend forward at waist, reaching elbows as close to floor as possible. Count 2. Return to starting position.

4.   KNEE PUSHUP

Starting position: Lie on floor, face down, legs together, knees bent with feet raised off floor, hands on floor under shoulders, palms down.

Action: Count 1. Push upper body off floor until arms are fully flexed and body in straight line from head to knees. Count 2. Return to starting position.

5.   SITUP (ARMS EXTENDED, KNEES UP)

Starting position: Lie on back, legs straight, arms extended overhead.
Action: Count 1. Sit up, reaching forward with arms encircling knees while pulling them tightly to chest. Count 2. Return to starting position. Do this exercise rhythmically, without breaks in the movement.

6.   LEG RAISER

Starting position: Right side of body on floor, head resting on right arm.

Action: Lift left leg about 24″ off floor, then lower it. Do required number of repetitions. Repeat on other side.

WOMEN: LEVEL THREE

Warmup Exercises	Exercises 1-6 of Orientation program

Conditioning Exercises	Uninterrupted repetitions
1. Toe touch	20
2. Sprinter	16

3. Sitting stretch (fingers laced) 15
4. Knee pushup...............................20
5. Situp (arms extended, knees up) 15
6. Leg raiser .... 16 each leg
7. Flutter kick...............................40

Circulatory activity (choose one each workout)

Jog-walk (jog 50, walk 50) ....¾ mile
Rope (skip 45 secs., rest 30 secs.) .... 3 series
Run in place .... 4 minutes

Water activities—See recommendations on page 106.

Your progress record 1 2 3 4 5 6 7 8 9 10 11 12 13 14 15

Prove-out
workouts

Step test (pulse)

---

7. FLUTTER KICK

Starting position: Lie face down, hands tucked under thighs.

Action: Arch the back, bringing chest and head up. Then flutter kick continuously, moving the legs 8"—10" apart. Kick from hips with knees slightly bent. Count each kick as one.

CIRCULATORY ACTIVITIES

JOG-WALK—Jog and walk alternately for number of paces indicated on chart for distance specified.

ROPE—Skip or jump rope continuously using any form for 45 seconds and then rest 30 seconds. Repeat 3 times.

RUN IN PLACE—Raise each foot at least 4" off floor and jog in place. Count 1 each time left foot touches floor. Complete number of running steps called for in chart, then do specified number of straddle hops. Complete number of running steps called for in chart, then do specified number of straddle hops. Complete 2 cycles of alternate running and hopping for time specified on chart.

STRADDLE HOP—Starting position: At attention.
Action: Count 1. Swing arms sideward and upward, touching hands above head (arms straight) while simultaneously moving feet sideward and apart in a single jumping motion. Count 2. Spring back to starting position. Two counts in one hop.

1. TOE TOUCH (TWIST AND BEND)

Starting position: Stand, feet shoulder-width apart, arms extended overhead, thumbs interlocked.

Action: Count 1. Twist trunk to right and touch floor inside right foot with fingers of both hands. Count 2. Touch floor outside toes of right foot. Count 3. Touch floor outside heel of right foot. Count 4. Return to starting position, sweeping trunk and arms upward in a wide arc. On the next four counts, repeat action to left side.

2. SPRINTER

Starting position: Squat, hands on floor, fingers pointed

forward, left leg fully extended to rear.

Action: Count 1. Reverse position of feet in bouncing movement, bringing left foot to hands, extending right leg backward—all in one motion. Count 2. Reverse feet again, returning to starting position.

3. SITTING STRETCH (ALTERNATE)

Starting position: Sit, legs spread apart, fingers laced behind neck, elbows back.

Action: Count 1. Bend forward to left, touching forehead to left knee. Count 2. Return to starting position. Count 3 and 4. Repeat to right. Score one repetition each time you return to starting position. Knees may be bent if necessary.

4. PUSHUP

Starting position: Lie on floor, face down, legs together, hands on floor under shoulders with fingers pointing straight ahead.

Action: Count 1. Push body off floor by extending arms so that weight rests on hands and toes. Count 2. Lower the body until chest touches floor.
Note: Body should be kept straight, buttocks should not be raised, abdomen should not sag.

5. SITUP (ARMS CROSSED, KNEES BENT)

Starting position: Lie on back, arms crossed on chest, hands grasping opposite shoulders, knees bent to right angle, feet flat on floor.

Action: Count 1. Curl up to sitting position. Count 2. Return to starting position.

6. LEG RAISER (WHIP)

Starting position: Right side of body on floor, right arm supporting head.

Action: Whip left leg up and down rapidly lifting as high as possible off the floor. Count each whip as one. Reverse position and whip right leg up and down.

WOMEN: LEVEL FOUR

Warmup Exercises	Exercises 1-6 of Orientation program

Conditioning Exercises	Uninterrupted repetitions
1. Toe touch (twist and bend)	5 each side
2. Springer	20
3. Sitting stretch (alternate)	20
4. Pushup	8
5. Situp (arms crossed, knees bent)	20
6. Leg raiser	10 each leg
7. Prone arch (arms extended)	15

Circulatory activity (choose one each workout)

Jog-walk (jog 100, walk 50)	1 mile
Rope (skip 60 secs., rest 30 secs.)	3 series
Run in place (run 145, hop 25 - 2 cycles	5 minutes

Water activities—See recommendations on page 106.

Step test (pulse)

7. PRONE ARCH (ARMS EXTENDED)

Starting position: Lie face down, legs straight and together, arms extended to sides at shoulder level.
Action: Count 1. Arch the back, bringing arms, chest and head up, and raising legs as high as possible. Count 2. Return to starting position.

CIRCULATORY ACTIVITIES

JOG—WALK—Jog and walk alternately for number of paces indicated on chart for distance specified.
ROPE—Skip or jump rope continuously using any form for 60 seconds and then rest 30 seconds. Repeat 3 times.
RUN IN PLACE—Raise each foot at least 4″ off floor and jog in place. Count 1 each time left foot touches floor. Complete number of running steps called for in chart, then do specified number of straddle hops. Complete 2 cycles of alternate running and hopping for time specified on chart.
STRADDLE HOP—Starting position: At attention.
    Action: Count 1. Swing arms sideward and upward, touching hands above head (arms straight) while simultaneously moving feet sideward and apart in a single jumping motion. Count 2. Spring back to starting position. Two counts in one hop.

1. TOE TOUCH (TWIST AND BEND)
Starting position: Stand, feet shoulder-width apart, arms extended overhead, thumbs interlocked.

Action: Count 1. Twist trunk to right and touch floor inside right foot with fingers of both hands. Count 2. Touch floor outside toes of right foot. Count 3. Touch floor outside heel of right foot. Count 4. Return to starting position, sweeping trunk and arms upward in a wide arc. On the next four counts, repeat action to left side.

2. SPRINTER

Starting position: Squat, hands on floor, fingers pointed forward, left leg fully extended to rear.
Action: Count 1. Reverse position of feet in bouncing movement, bringing left foot to hands and extending right leg backward—all in one motion. Count 2. Reverse feet again, returning to starting position.

3. SITTING STRETCH (ALTERNATE)

Starting position: Sit, legs spread apart, fingers behind neck, elbows back.
Action: Count 1. Bend forward to left, touching forehead to left knee. Count 2. Return to starting position. Counts 3 and 4. Repeat to right. Score one repetition each time you return to starting position. Knees may be bent if necessary.

4. PUSHUP

Starting position: Lie on floor, face down, legs together, hands on floor under shoulders with fingers pointing straight ahead.
Action: Count 1. Push body off floor by extending arms so that weight rests on hands and toes. Count 2. Lower the body until chest touches floor.

Note: Body should be kept straight, buttocks should not be raised, abdomen should not sag.

5. SITUP (FINGERS LACED, KNEES BENT)

Starting position: Lie on back, fingers laced behind neck, knees bent, feet flat on floor.
Action: Count 1. Sit up, turn trunk to right, touch left elbow to right knee. Count 2. Return to starting position. Count 3. Sit up, turn trunk to left, touch right elbow to left knee. Count 4. Return to starting position. Score one each time you return to starting position.

6. LEG RAISER

Starting position: Lie on right side, body rigidly supported by extended right arm and foot. Left arm is held behind head.
Action: Count 1. Raise left leg high. Count 2. Return to starting position slowly. Repeat on other side. Do required number of repetitions.

WOMEN: LEVEL FIVE

Warmup Exercises	Exercises 1-6 of Orientation program

Conditioning Exercises	Uninterrupted repetitions
1. Toe touch (twist and bend)	25 each side
2. Sprinter	24
3. Sitting stretch (alternate)	26
4. Pushup	15
5. Situp (fingers laced, knees bent)	25
6. Leg raiser (on extended arm)	10 each side
7. Prone arch (fingers laced)	25

Circulatory activity (choose one each workout)

Jog-run . . . . 1 mile
Rope (skip 2 mins, rest 45 sec.) . . . . 2 series
Run in place (run 180, hop 30 - 2 cycles) . . . 6 minutes

Water activities—See recommendations on page 106.

Your progress record 1 2 3 4 5 6 7 8 9 10 11 12 13 14 15
Prove-out
workouts

Step test (pulse)

7. PRONE ARCH (FINGERS LACED)
Starting position: Lie face down, fingers laced behind neck.

Action: Count 1. Arch back, legs and chest off floor. Count 2. Extend arms fully forward. Count 3. Return hands to behind neck. Count 4. Flatten body to floor.

CIRCULATORY ACTIVITIES

JOG-RUN—Jog and run alternately for distance specified on chart.

ROPE—Skip or jump rope continuously using any form for 2 minutes and then rest 45 seconds. Repeat 2 times.

RUN IN PLACE—Raise each foot at least 4″ off floor and jog in place. Count 1 each time left foot touches floor. Complete number of running steps called for in chart, then do specified number of straddle hops. Complete 2 cycles of alternate running and hopping in time specified on the chart.

STRADDLE HOP—Starting position: At attention.

Action: Count 1. Swing arms sideward and upward, touching hands above head (arms straight) while simultaneously moving feet sideward and apart in a single jumping motion. Count 2. Spring back to starting position. Two counts in one hop.

Staying fit
Once you have reached the level of conditioning you have chosen for yourself, you will wish to maintain your fitness.

To do so, continue the workouts at that level.

While it has been found possible to maintain fitness with three workouts a week, ideally, exercise should be a daily habit. If you can, by all means continue your workouts on a five-times-a-week basis.

If at any point—either after reaching your goal or in the process of doing so—your workouts are interrupted because of illness or other reason for more than a week, it will be best to begin again at a lower level. If you have had a serious illness or surgery, proceed under your physician's guidance.

Broadening your program
The exercises and activities you have engaged in are basic—designed to take you soundly and progressively up the ladder to physical fitness without need for special equipment or facilities.

There are many other activities and forms of exercise which, if you wish, you may use to supplement the basic program. You will find them discussed in the following sections. They include a variety of sports; water exercises you can use if you have access to a pool; and isometrics—

sometimes called exercises without movement—which take little time (6-8 seconds each).One isometric—the abdominal—is particularly valuable for many women; it helps strengthen muscles that can act like a girdle to maintain a trim waistline.

You'll find suggestions, too, for improving posture—and also for taking advantage of many daily opportunities for sound physical activity.

DAILY OPPORTUNITIES FOR ADDING TO FITNESS

There are many—and, by taking advantage of them, you can speed your progress to—and more easily maintain—your top level of fitness.

Here are some examples:

Stairs—versus elevators or escalator: At least now and then, choose the stairs. And bound up them—take two at a time as often as possible.

Breaks—Along with, or instead of, those midmorning and midafternoon time-outs for coffee, take exercise breaks. No need to get into a sweat. Do a conditioning exercise or two if convenient. If you lack privacy, do some of the inconspicuous isometric exercises.

Pull-ins—suck in your abdomen now and then, hold it taut for a few seconds.

Up for a stretch—if you must work in static, sitting position, get up occasionally, stand erect, stretch a bit, move around.

Rub away—after a shower or bath, towel yourself vigorously. That's exercise, too—stimulating for muscles as well as skin.

Walking deserves special emphasis

Walking is actually one of the best all-round physical activities. The massaging action the leg muscles exert on the veins as you walk improves the flow of blood back to the heart; when you walk you're improving not only your leg muscles but also the pumping action they provide. Walking costs nothing; there are many possible daily opportunities for it, and it can be enjoyable. Develop a brisk step, breathe deeply, swing your arms.

Allow extra time to get to the train, to the store, to meetings, other places you have to go so you can go, at least now and then, by footpower.

Whenever you feel tense and nervous, try a walk—the brisker and longer, the better, but even a brief one will help discharge tension. Use a before-bed walk as an aid to sleep; it can be a big help in overcoming insomnia.

On an occasional weekend, plan walking as a family enterprise. Set a goal; take a walking tour to a park, other scenic spot, or some place of historical interest.

Whenever possible, adults should join physical fitness groups conducted under professional supervision. Such classes are available at local clubs, churches, schools, colleges, community recreation centers, and at the Y's and other voluntary agencies.

ISOMETRICS

Isometric contraction exercises take very little time, require no special equipment. They're excellent muscle strengtheners and, as such, valuable supplements.

The idea of isometrics is to work out a muscle by pushing or pulling against an immovable object such as a wall...or by pitting it against the opposition of another muscle.

The basis is the "overload" principle of exercise physiology—which holds that a muscle required to perform work beyond the usual intensity will grow in strength. And research has been indicating that one hard, 6-8-second isometric contraction per workout can, over a period of six months, significantly increase muscle strength.

The exercises described in the following pages cover major large muscle groups of the body.

They can be performed almost anywhere and at almost any time.

There is no set order for doing them—nor do all have to be completed at one time. You can, if you like, do one or two in the morning, others at various times during the day whenever you have half a minute or even less to spare.

For each contraction, maintain tension *no more than eight seconds*. Do little breathing during a contraction; breathe deeply between contractions.

And start easily. Do *not* apply maximum effort in the beginning.

For the first three or four weeks, you should exert only about one-half what you think is your maximum force.

Use the first three or four seconds to build up to this degree of force—and the remaining four or five seconds to hold it.

For the next two weeks, gradually increase force to more nearly approach maximum. After about six weeks, it will be safe to exert maximum effort.

Pain indicates you're applying too much force; reduce the

amount immediately. If pain continues to accompany any exercise, discontinue using that exercise for a week or two. Then try it again with about 50 percent of maximum effort and, if no pain occurs, you can go on to gradually build up toward maximum.

NECK
Starting position: Sit or stand, with interlaced fingers of hands on forehead.
Action: Forcibly exert a forward push of head while resisting equally hard with hands.
Starting position: Sit or stand, with interlaced fingers or hands behind head.
Action: Push head backward while exerting a forward pull with hands.
Starting position: Sit or stand, with palm of left hand on left side of head.
Action: Push with left hand while resisting with head and neck.
Reverse using right hand on right side of head.

UPPER BODY
Starting position: Stand, back to wall, hands at sides, palms toward wall.
Action: Press hands backward against wall, keeping arms straight.
Starting position: Stand, facing wall, hands at sides, palms toward wall.
Action: Press hands forward against wall, keeping arms straight.
Starting position: Stand in doorway or with side against wall, arms at sides, palms toward legs.
Action: Press hand(s) outward against wall or doorframe, keeping arms straight.

ARMS
Starting position: Stand with feet slightly apart. Flex

right elbow, close to body, palm up. Place left hand over right.

Action: Forcibly attempt to curl right arm upward, while giving equally strong resistance with the left hand. Repeat with left arm.

Starting position: Stand with feet comfortably spaced, knees slightly bent. Clasp hands, palms together, close to chest.

Action: Press hands together and hold.

Starting position: Stand with feet slightly apart, knees slightly bent. Grip fingers, arms close to chest.

Action: Pull hard and hold.

ABDOMINAL
Starting position: Stand, knees slightly flexed, hands resting on knees.

Action: Contract abdominal muscles.

LOWER BACK, BUTTOCKS AND BACKS OF THIGHS
Starting position: Lie face down, arms at sides, palms up, legs placed under bed or other heavy object.

Action: With both hips flat on floor, raise one leg, keeping knee straight so that heel pushes hard against the resistance above. Repeat with opposite leg.

LEGS
Starting position: Sit in chair with left ankle crossed over right, feet resting on floor, legs bent a 90 degree angle.

Action: Forcibly attempt to straighten right leg while resisting with the left. Repeat with opposite leg.

INNER AND OUTER THIGHS
Starting position: Sit, legs extended with each ankle pressed against the outside of sturdy chair legs.

Action: Keep legs straight and pull toward one another firmly. For outer thigh muscles, place ankles inside chair legs and exert pressure outward.

WATER ACTIVITIES

Swimming is one of the best physical activities for people of all ages—and for many of the handicapped.

With the body submerged in water, blood circulation automatically increases to some extent; pressure of water on the body also helps promote deeper ventilation of the lungs; and with well-planned activity, both circulation and ventilation increase still more.

The water exercises described on the following page can be used either as supplements to, or replacements for, the circulatory activities of the basic program. The goals for each of the five levels are shown in the chart below.

WOMEN

Level	1	2	3	4	5
Bobs	10	15	20	50	100
Swim	5 min	10 min	15 min		
Interval swimming				25 yds. (Repeat 10 times)	25 yds. (Repeat 20 times)

BOBBING

Starting position: Face out of water

Action: Count 1. Take a breath. Count 2. Submerge while exhaling until feet touch bottom. Count 3. Push up from bottom to surface while continuing to exhale. Three counts to one bob.

SWIMMING

Use any type of stroke. Swim continuously for the time specified.

INTERVAL SWIMMING

Use any type of stroke. Swim moderately fast for distance specified. You can then either swim back slowly to starting point or get out of pool and walk back. Repeat specified number of times.

WEIGHT TRAINING

Weight training also is an excellent method of developing muscular strength—and muscular endurance. Where equipment is available, it may be used as a supplement to the seven conditioning exercises.

Because of the great variety of weight training exercises, there will be no attempt to describe them here. Both barbells and weighted dumbbells—complete with instructions—are available at most sporting goods stores. A good rule to follow in deciding the maximum weight you should lift is to select a weight you can lift six times without strain.

SPORTS

Soccer, basketball, handball, squash, ice hockey and other sports that require sustained effort can be valuable aids to building circulatory endurance.

But if you have been sedentary, it's important to pace yourself carefully in such sports, and it may even be advisable to avoid them until you are well along in your physical conditioning program. That doesn't mean you should avoid all sports.

There are many excellent conditioning and circulatory activities in which the amount of exertion is easily controlled and in which you can progress at your own rate. Bicycling is one example. Others include hiking, skating, tennis, running, cross-country skiing, rowing, canoeing, water skiing and skindiving. You can engage in these sports at any point in the program, if you start slowly. Games should be played with full speed and vigor only when your conditioning permits doing so without undue fatigue.

On days when you get a good workout in sports you can skip part or all of your exercise program. Use your own judgment.

If you have engaged in a sport which exercises the legs and stimulates the heart and lungs—such as skating—you could skip the circulatory activity for that day, but you still should do some of the conditioning and stretching exercises for the upper body. On the other hand, weightlifting is an excellent conditioning activity, but it should be supplemented with running or one of the other circulatory exercises.

Whatever your favorite sport, you will find your enjoyment enhanced by improved fitness. Every weekend athlete should invest in frequent workouts.

POSTURE

There is a relationship between good posture and physical fitness—one helps the other.

Good posture acts to avoid cramping of internal organs, permits better circulation, prevents undue tensing of some muscles and undue lengthening of others. It thus contributes to fitness.

In turn, physical conditioning, by developing muscle tone, helps to make good posture more readily maintainable—and will help, too, if you have any bad postural habits you need to break.

For good posture, the centers of gravity of many body parts—feet, legs, hips, trunk, shoulders and head—must be in a vertical line. As viewed from the side when you are standing, the line should run through ear lobe, tip of shoulder, middle of hips, just back of kneecap, just in front of outer ankle bone.

Proper posture positions are:

STANDING: 1. Feet parallel, about 6″ apart. 2. Head high, as if balancing a book. 3. Chest out. 4. Stomach and hips firm. 5. Abdomen and back as flat as possible. 6. Knees very lightly flexed—not stiffly locked. 7. Weight evenly distributed on both feet—most of it on balls of feet.

SITTING

1. Sit tall and back, with hips touching the back of the chair, feet flat on floot. 2. Chest out, back of neck nearly in line with upper back. 3. When writing, lean forward from the hips so you keep head and shoulders in line.

WALKING

1. Knees and ankles limber, toes pointed straight ahead. 2. Head and chest high. 3. Swing legs directly forward from hip joints. 4. Push feet off the ground—don't shuffle. 5. Swing shoulders and arms freely and easily.

The position of the hips is one reliable indicator of posture. They should rest squarely upon the legs without tilting forward or backward.

Flabby abdominal muscles and excess weight—

particularly in the abdominal region—are frequent causes of poor posture. Weak abdominal muscles permit the internal organs to drop. The results: the abdomen protrudes, the pelvis tilts forward and the curve of the lower back is accentuated. Lower back pains may occur.

The obese person's "paunch" upsets his center of gravity. As it pulls him forward he compensates by leaning backward, bending his knees slightly and increasing the curve of his back. This produces the characteristic "old man's stance."

Excessive use of high-heeled shoes can produce the same effect in women—even young women. Additionally, the muscles in the calves and the backs of the thighs are shortened, so that it may be uncomfortable to go barefoot or wear low heels.

Forward head, or "poked neck," is another common posture fault. When the head is out of line, some other part of the body compensates and also moves out of line. Get the "feel" of proper posture positions. Practice them until they become habitual.

Exercising in a Group

If you find it hard to maintain a physical-fitness program all by yourself, you're not alone. Successful groups such as Weight Watchers started because people discovered that what was next-to-impossible to accomplish as a single person was much easier with the support of a group. When I was still struggling with what had been a weight problem, I knew the only way to stay in shape for the rest of my life was to make a commitment to exercise for the rest of my life. Along with some of my friends—many of them well-known business and professional women—I formed a group so that we could all give each other the help and support so lacking when you try to maintain physical fitness all alone.

For many women a woman's group is the best place to find sympathetic friends with similar problems and goals. Some people, however, find the ideal exercise partner is the husband or lover with whom they share so many other areas of life. Since exercise is such a large part of life, I take advantage of both.

One of the advantages to exercising either with a group at a health club or with your husband at home is that the program continues winter and summer, no matter what the weather. And if you have an arrangement with at least one other person, you're much less likely to backslide, to let it go "just for today," because you got home late from the office or have a headache. If you decide to work out a program with your husband, be sure to pick a certain time of day—every day—and then stick to it. If you belong to a club, you'll probably sign up for a specific time for exercise classes. Midday is an ideal time, and very possible if you join a club that's near your home or office. It's usually not so likely that you'll be able to get together with your spouse at lunchtime, so most couples, including my husband and me, exercise between dinner and bedtime. Don't wait until just before you're ready to go to sleep, though, because exercise is too stimulating to be a good pre-bed routine.

The exercises I do with my husband are especially designed for two people to do co-operatively. But you can, if you choose, do separate exercises—together only in that the two of you work out in the same room at the same time. The factor of moral support will still be with you. Remember to take into account when you exercise in any group, that there will be initial differences in stamina and ability. That's particularly true when you exercise with your husband, especially if he's already in good condition. A group may help urge you on to do just a little bit more, but don't be shy about quitting when you get really tired. The idea is to get in shape gradually, not knock yourself out in one session.

Chapter VI:
Dieting Made Simple

In its broad outlines, the problem really is simple. If you take in more calories than you expend, you'll get fat. Of course, that's something like saying that economics is a simple matter of taking in as much as you pay out; it's simple on the outside, very complex when you get down to nitty gritty analysis. Most people do not want to go on diets that require them to become instant nutritionists, biochemists, or home economists. They like to have the facts explained to them, yes, but they also like to have the diet planning done by the experts.

The facts, then, are these. Calories *do* count, but they count in different ways at different times. So much depends on your habits and your metabolism, plus your age and nutritional needs. You can eat 1,000 calories a day of Danish pastry and chocolate chips, and you'll probably lose weight. You'll also wind up undernourished, sugar-freaked, and badly in need of some heavy dental work. You can eat 1,000 calories a day of vegetables, lose weight, and suffer from a protein deficiency. Or you can eat 1,000 calories a day of *different* vegetables in the right combinations, lose weight, and remain perfectly healthy. Some people can lose weight on close to 2,000 calories a day. Others, the small and slight, have to drop down to about 700 to get the weight-loss program underway. You can lose weight eating pounds of steak a day, but you run the risk of tipping your body chemistry off balance, not to mention your budget.

Never underestimate the psychological factor in diet. One woman had such a hard time sticking to any diet that I recommended a doctor friend of mine. It seemed like time for her to have a complete physical and see if there was any organic reason why she couldn't lose weight. This is what the doctor reported to me: "I checked this woman over and she seemed absolutely normal. Thirty-five and in good health—I couldn't think of any good reason why she couldn't get thin. So I have her a standard 1200-calorie diet, but she wouldn't even look at it. She said she wanted something new, the latest innovation. She said she already knew the standard diet wouldn't work for her. So I said, just out of the blue, 'Eat three oranges every day, a small salad with cheese at lunch, and a bran-and-banana milkshake for dinner. Once a week have steak.' Three weeks later she came back saying, 'Doctor, the Orange Diet is fabulous—I've lost 14 pounds!'" The doctor's analysis was that as long as the lady thought she was using the "latest thing," she had enough motivation to stick it out and lose weight. She just couldn't stand to be one of the herd using the same old moderate diet as everyone else.

I think some of the same principles are operating behind all the very simple fad diets such as Dr. Stillman, Dr. Atkins, and the Scarsdale Diet. There are very few foods allowed on these diets, so it's easy to remember what you have to do. No indecision ever results, because you don't get to make any decisions. Plus, there's the satisfaction of knowing you're using the newest techniques. Not that I think there's anything wrong with any of these regimens, including the Orange Diet, for brief periods. But my doctor friend and I agree that to really lose weight and keep it off, you need to change your pattern of eating for good, not just for two or three weeks.

If you use a quick-loss fad diet to begin your program, you might as well realize right now that it's only a start. It may boost your morale to lose a few pounds fast, and give you incentive to work on the slower, longer process of re-vamping your whole attitude toward food. But the latter task must be undertaken if you want to avoid the yo-yo syndrome that afflicts so many, many dieters.

Let me say right here that everyone, no matter what your age, should check with your doctor before going on a diet. That's just in case you have some metabolic oddity or health problem that would make an ordinarily harmless diet detrimental to your well-being. Probably, you're just fine, but it never hurts to be sure. But be prepared to take the advice you pay for. If the physician says a high-protein, low-carbohydrate diet is not for you, for example, don't go against him. If you insist on undermining your health just to be fashionably skinny, you stand a very good chance of being too ill to enjoy your new svelteness. Another time you should see a doctor: if you're more than 20 pounds overweight. Most people have, like me, ten pounds or so that have a way of sneaking back on from time to time. We're always trying eight to shed those Big Ten or to keep them off the easy way by staying active and never eating any chocolate sundaes. But if your weight problem is more substantial than ours, you're going to have to commit yourself to a long-term regimen. And for that, you really should have the advice of a medical person, as well as a checkup.

The Basic Makeover Diet I'll give you in this chapter includes no crutches. Though it's a good idea to take a multi-vitamin tablet every day, it isn't necessary on this diet, because it's completely nutritionally balanced. You don't have to gulp grapefruit juice and you must not take diuretics or stimulants. These are hard drugs, and safe only by prescription. Even then, I'd say proceed with caution. Some people react very badly to amphetamine-type diet pills, just as do kids who take them illicitly. If you're in the habit of relying on diet pills and the "high" they give you that lets you race through the day without eating, let me tell you a secret: reducing your caloric intake can provide a very similar high, all by itself. That's why people like Jane Fonda call fasting a "natural stimulant." Generally speaking, and the reasons are probably traced to evolution, being slightly food-deprived makes you more alert, more lively. It stands to reason that that reaction would be good for survival, since an alert and hungry animal is more likely to find food than a lethargic and hungry one. Try two or three days of my Makeover Diet, with no pills, and see if you don't get something of the same feeling as with amphetamines, but much more controlled and ever so much safer.

Fasting

Since we've mentioned it, it might as well be said: fasting is very hard on the body. Yes, you can do it and survive. The human race would have died long ago if that weren't the case. But it's an extreme state, and one that causes the body's normal biochemical mechanisms to go into reverse, in a sense, burning what is normally used for other purposes. Part of what's burned is your muscle tissue—and that can happen before the fat is used up. The body needs protein all the time, and if you're not supplying it from the outside, your body will "cannibalize" its own tissues to get it. So you may end up reducing what you want to keep and keeping the pads of fat you want to get rid of. The above-quoted Ms. Fonda says she fasts for two or three days before every new undertaking to "clear out the system," and get herself in a euphoric frame of mind. In a person with sound health (see your doctor), two or three days probably won't hurt anything. But prolonged fasting is for the fanatic and the desperate. One of the positive lessons to be learned from fasting, I think, is just how much of our lives revolve around the procurement, preparation, consuming, and just contemplating of food. A friend of mine who went on a short fast said she didn't know what to do with all the time she suddenly had on her hands. If you've ever been pressed for time, *and* you'd like to take off a few pounds, you might take a tip from my friend's experience. You don't have to be on a fast to de-emphasize the food ritual.

Ketosis

Ketosis is the name for the biochemical state your body gets in when you take in surplus protein but not enough carbohydrate. The Dr. Atkins diet uses the ketotic state to diagnose whether or not the dieter is doing it right. On that diet, ketosis is synonymous with the weight-loss process. Since ketosis in a clinical setting has traditionally been the symptom of disease, often of serious illness, doctors are naturally wary of any process that intentionally induces what is thought of as a pathological condition. The best part of the low-low carbohydrate diets is that you never feel hungry, though you might feel a little sick from all that hard-to-digest fat and meat sitting on your stomach. The bad part is that there is much controversy over whether or not the ketotic diets are harmful to your health. It would be a shame to discover, too late, that this extreme weight-loss program had done damage to your bodily well-being. Also, Dr. Atkins' diet makes your breath smell fruity.

Calories

Even the most simplified diet plan has to include the rudiments of calorie arithmetic, so here goes: a pound of fat is worth 3,500 calories. That's how much you have to cut out of your diet to lose one pound. Most of us can't lose a pound a day because we don't take in 3,500 calories a day in the first place. Even if we cut down to nothing, we won't consistently lose a pound a day. It's true that if you step up your activity you can burn more calories than normal and speed up your weight loss, but the arithmetic remains the same. A rough calculation of how many calories you should have in your reducing diet can be obtained by multiplying your ideal weight by 10. If you'd like to weigh 120, for instance, you should be eating about 1200 calories a day. Since this is roughly the average ideal weight for the American woman, the 1200-calorie diet is the most popular for small-boned women. If you truly have a large frame—but watch out, lots more women think they have big bones than really do—1600 calories a day is more like it for you. The average person, of whatever frame, can lose a pound a week on 2000 calories, if—and it's a big if—she can stick with it long enough. But most of us need quicker results, or we get demoralized.

Liquid Protein

This stuff looks and tastes like rancid cough syrup and is made from old cow hides. You're supposed to drink it on a modified-fast diet to keep your body from using its muscle-protein. Since there are a good number of serious questions concerning the safety of this product and the diet, I doubt that you can buy liquid protein much anymore. If you do see a bottle, leave it on the shelf.

Diet Soda

A wonderful invention that has been shrouded by doubts about the safety of artificial sweeteners ever since the cyclamate controversy. The latest word, to my great delight, is that tests have shown that saccharin will not cause cancer in humans in the amounts ingested by the average person or even the average dieter. In all likelihood, there's nothing very healthy in diet soda except the water. Besides artificial color, flavor, and sweeteners, it contains caffeine and carbonation. Drinking too much will produce reactions in most people very like their reactions to too much coffee. Used in moderation, however, there's nothing like it to take the edge off a diet and keep you from feeling like a martyr to the cause of skinniness. Use it as a special treat for yourself when you've been extra good. But watch out you don't generalize the practice so you start rewarding yourself with sugar when the diet is over.

Cooking

Lots of people complain that what they hate most about dieting is having to spend the same amount of time or even more in the kitchen. "If I'm not supposed to dwell on food," as one woman put it, "how come this diet has me hovering over the stove all the time?" Other women, who have to cook for their non-dieting families, are tempted unmercifully by dishes their husbands and children can have, but they can't. When this question comes up, I always tell the women this: "On my diet, there's nothing that isn't good for your whole family. All the meals are well-balanced and nutritionally sound. There's no reason your husband and children can't have the same thing you're having, though maybe their portions will be larger. Besides, this is a good way to improve their eating habits—get them off rich sauces and fried foods." All the meats on my diet are broiled, boiled, or baked—with no added grease. And the meals are all simple—easy and quick to prepare, even if you're cooking for a whole crowd.

I can sympathize with people who patronize those diet services that actually provide the meals for you—you go down every day or once a week and they give you everything you're allowed to eat in a grocery bag. Of course it's easier to stay on the diet, at least for a while, if you don't have to think about it. But dieting, just like exercise, is forever. Either you're going to form good eating habits now, or you're going to be back on the diet a few weeks or months from now. My preferred diet, the one I'm going to put you on for your 14-Day Makeover, is as conservative as it can be. It also works, not just in the short run, but in the long haul, too.

Meals

As you'll see right away, my diet calls for a breakfast, a lunch and a dinner. I want you to meat them all, even if you're in the habit of skipping breakfast or lunch and "saving up" for dinner. On no account must you eat any other meals. Dieters usually tell me that late nights—the period after dinner—are the worst times. And I know from my own battle of the bulge (I went from a size 14 to a size 7) that they're right. The solution that works best for me is to find something else to do, something that's incompatible with eating. On nights when you have theater tickets, it's easy enough. But if you want to get thin and stay thin, I think you have to give up the midnight snack forever, even if the only alternative you can think of is going to sleep early. It might not strike you as thrilling, but it's good for you, and it'll put you in better shape to take advantage of the big nights when they do come along.

About breakfast: many people have told me that the very idea of eating in the morning makes them feel ill. I say that's probably because they stayed up late, stuffing themselves. I've never known a little child who was not a "morning person" and who didn't start each day eager for all kinds of experience, including breakfast. Somehow, as we get older, we get into a rhythm where we start slower and slower in the mornings, and it's only aggravated by skipping breakfast. That means you have no fuel to run through the morning on, and that's after six to eight hours of enforced fasting while you were asleep. No wonder some people don't seem to wake up until the afternoon—that's the first time there's any nourishment in their bloodstreams.

The ideal spacing of meals is about 5½ to 6 hours apart. Most of us can't quite manage that, so we eat our breakfast and lunch closer together and wait longer for dinner. That's all right, as long as your meals are roughly equidistant and you maintain a regular pattern. Of course, I don't care what time you eat the meals, but most of us who work during the day have to eat at about 8 a.m., 12 p.m., and 7 p.m., with dinner being the most flexible meal. If you're an actress who works half the night and sleeps half the day, you'll have to adjust your pattern accordingly. But whatever time it is when it's "morning" for you, be sure to eat a good breakfast.

The Diet

Here it is, pure and simple as it can be. Follow this diet every day of your 14-Day Makeover, and you'll lose from 2 to 4 pounds a week. Best of all, you can stay on this diet as long as you need to to reach your ideal weight. It's not the kind that will make you sick if you follow it more than two weeks.

Breakfast

Fruit—Choose ONE from the list below

Protein Food-Choose ONE: 2 oz. cottage or pot cheese
2 oz. cooked or canned fish
1 egg (no more than 4 eggs a week)

Bread or Cereal (enriched or whole grain) 1 slice bread OR

3/4 cup ready-to-eat cereal
or 1/2 cup cooked cereal
WITH SKIM MILK

Coffee or Tea, no milk or sugar. Artificial sweetener may be used.

Lunch

Protein Food—Choose ONE: 2 oz. fish, poultry or lean meat
4 oz. cottage or pot cheese
2 oz. hard cheese (No more than twice a week.)

Bread, enriched or whole grain: 2 slices
Vegetables-raw or cooked—all you want except potato or substitute.
Fruit—any kind—small serving, no sugar.
Coffee or Tea.

Dinner

Protein Food—Choose ONE: 4 oz cooked lean meat, poultry, or fish.
Vegetables—raw: 1 high vitamin A (see below)
   raw or cooked: Potato or Substitute (see below
Other vegetables: all you want

Fruit—any kind—small serving, no sugar
Coffee or Tea.

Fat: Choose ONE from the list below.

Milk: 2 cups of skim milk or substitute from the list below.

High Vitamin C Fruits
4 oz. unsweetened orange or grapefruit juice
1/2 medium grapefruit
1/2 cup strawberries
1 large tangerine
1 medium orange
8 oz. tomato juice
1 medium mango

1 small guava
1/2 medium cantaloupe
1/2 small papaya

High Vitamin A Vegetables

Broccoli
Carrots
Chicory
Collards
Dandelion greens
Escarole
Kale

Mustard greens
Pumpkin
Spinach
Swiss Chard
Turnip greens
Watercress
Winter squash

Potato or Substitute

1 medium potato
1 small sweet potato or yam
½ cup corn
½ cup cooked dry beans, peas, or lentils
½ cup green peas
½ cup lima beans
½ cup cooked rice, spaghetti, macaroni, grits, or noodles
½ cup plantain

Fat

1 Tablespoon vegetable oil
1 Tablespoon mayonnaise
1 Tablespoon margarine with liquid vegetable oil listed first on the label
2 Tablespoons French dressing

Skim Milk or Substitute

2 cups (8 oz. each) fat-free liquid skim milk or buttermilk
1 cup (8 oz.) skimmed evaporated milk
2/3 cup instant nonfat dry milk

1. You may Drink:
Coffee
Tea
Water

Seltzer
Bouillon
Consomme

2. You may Use:

Salt	Spices
Pepper	Horseradish
Herbs	Lemon, lime

3. You May Have as Snacks:
Vegetables—raw or cooked—all you want

Asparagus	Lettuce
Green beans	Mushrooms
Broccoli	Mustard Greens
Brussels Sprouts	Parsley
Cabbage	Pimiento
Carrots	Romaine
Cauliflower	Spinach
Celery	Summer squash
Chicory	Swiss Chard
Collards	Tomato
Dandelion greens	Tomato juice
Escarole	Turnip
Kale	Watercress

4. Do Not Eat or Drink:

Bacon, sausage	Jam, jelly
Beer, wine, liquor	Milk, whole
Butter, most margarine	Muffins
Cream, sweet & sour	Nuts
Cakes, cookies	Peanut butter
Candy	Olives
Crackers, bagels	Pancakes, waffles
Doughnuts	Pastries, pie
Gelatin desserts	Pizza
Gravy, sauces	Popcorn, pretzels
Ice cream, ices	Potato chips and similar
Sherbet	snack foods

Puddings	Syrup, honey
Soda	Yogurt
Sugar	

As you must have noticed, there's no drinking on this diet. I'm not one of those who thinks that a drink now and then or wine with a good dinner is bad for you, but I do think it plays havoc with dieters. Besides the calories, which are considerable for the small amount of space it takes up, alcohol interferes with judgment. If you went to an expensive spa for two weeks, they wouldn't let you drink, either. They know it makes you add calories and lose willpower, just the reverse of the intention of their program—and mine.

Your 14-Day Makeover

Exercise

Throughout the next two weeks, you'll be following the exercise program outlined in my chapter on exercise. Remember that even if you are doing the exercises for two with your man, you must also maintain a separate program of fitness just for yourself. After you've taken the test to determine your current fitness level, begin one of the series of exercises specified for your level. If you reach or surpass your goal, it's time to move up to the next level. I hope you'll be able to keep your exercise program going for five days a week, but even after the makeover sessions are over, exercising three times a week is an absolute minimum if you want to retain the benefits.

Diet

During your two-week makeover, you must follow my diet to the letter. The diet is one place where I allow no leeway at all. Women who are on a weight-loss diet should weigh themselves no more than once a week. I know it's hard to keep away from the scale, especially if you think you're doing well and want the rewarding sight of a smaller number in the little window. But so many factors can influence your weight from day to day—amount of fluid retained, for example—that the only way to get an accurate picture is to keep your weighings a week apart. You not only avoid false optimism that way, but false discouragement, too.

Daily Treat

Besides your regular diet and exercise—building good habits for the rest of your life—there's a different activity every day to help you re-organize your grooming techniques and streamline your looks. When you finish this two-week program, you'll not only be thinner and fitter, but you'll know how to highlight to advantage the radiant new you.

FIRST DAY

After you've had your breakfast, weighed in, and done your exercises, it's off to the hairdresser. Please plan your Makeover Program to begin on a day when you can take time to get a haircut, because it's so important to the success of the rest of the course that you start out on the right foot. I wish I could tell you how to give yourself a good, precise haircut. I wish I could tell myself! But I've interviewed several talented cutters on this point, and all of them told me the same thing: there's no way you—or they—can give a good haircut to the same head that owns the hands. A great cut involves a perspective, an artist's eye, that you just can't have when the hair you're cutting is your own. "Yes," said one top cutter, "its possible to cut your own hair. Just barely possible. I've seen those books that show you how to do it. But I'm sure of this, that it isn't possible to do it well. None of those books tells you how you're supposed to get *behind* your own head, and there's the rub." Lucky for hairdressers that they have each other to rely on—you know, "you cut mine and

I'll cut yours." But the rest of us, unless we have a haircutter in the family, have to pay. Look at it this way and it won't seem so bad: it's not only an investment in your future good looks, it's recreation. I don't know of anything more soothing, more luxurious, than having somebody wash your hair for you. And who else do you know who will happily discuss your face, your hair, your beauty needs without once mentioning his or her own? That's luxury, too.

The Cut

It's psychologically important where you get your cut, what the environment is like, whether you like the perfume they put in the air and the music. But the main thing is what they do to your hair, and the main thing they do to your hair is cut it. You've chosen a salon with a good reputation, one whose work you've seen and admired on friends. Maybe you have a personal recommendation to this cutter, or maybe it's your regular hairdresser whom you've known and trusted for years. Whatever the particulars, you're ready for the cut to begin.

As the cut proceeds, here are points to watch:
1. Does the cut begin on wet or dry hair? Unless your hairdresser has a very good reason, the cut should be done on wet hair. A few haircutters feel that certain kinds of hair—the very curly is the usual example—should be cut dry so that the cutter can see how the hair behaves in its normal state. But most hairdressers still say that there's no way to get the precision of line the discriminating client wants unless the hair is wet. Almost without exception, haircutters also prefer hair to be very, very clean. Unless it's just been washed fifteen minutes before you entered the salon, the good hairdresser will insist that you have a shampoo. Rarely is this an attempt to run up your bill. On the contrary, it's an attempt to be sure you'll be satisfied with the results instead of

disappointed.

2. Does the cutter consult you? I don't mean just at the beginning, when he or she says, "What kind of cut did you have in mind," but all through the process. A good haircutter doesn't have to keep any secrets from the client. Nor are they locked into a plan that admits no alterations once the cut has begun. If you don't like the way things seem to be going, if you think it's going to be too long in the back and too short on the sides, or if you know from experience that your bangs tend to curl so that they have to be cut a bit longer than usual, don't hesitate to say so. You'll never get an argument from a really great haircutter—they want to please you. Less talented people only have five or six stereotyped routines or cuts, and they get confused if you ask for anything the least bit different. (A good way to spot a novice is if he or she refers to what's being done to your hair as a "Model Cut," or a "Samantha," or some such moniker, instead of just "the cut." A cut from a good and experienced haircutter is unique—it's never just a cookie-cutter "Samantha" like everyone else's.

3. Does the cut proceed in an orderly way? A good cutter will carefully section your hair, snipping only one section at a time while the others are pinned up out of the way. Then, after each individual section has been done, they should be made to mesh smoothly with one another by a technique of cross-cutting. You may not be perfectly schooled in all the fine points, but you'll be able to tell, if you're paying attention, whether the job is being carefully done or if the cutter is snipping more or less at random around your head. The cut should proceed from the back to the sides to the top to the front, with bangs last.

4. The style. Probably, your hair will be dried either by blower or under a heat lamp. If you've asked for an

absolutely no-care style, it'll be the heat lamp. But beware of the stylist who insists he or she can give any kind of hair a drip-dry that never needs blowing or setting. These sorts of cuts have to be short, first of all, and they really only come out stunning on naturally curly hair of just the right texture. If you have really marvelous bones—but really marvelous—you can have your hair long and dry it in one of those twist-up to set styles, but since it may take hours to dry that way, such styles don't work well in the winter. For those who, like most women, have fine or thin or slightly-wavy-and-therefore-unruly hair, a touch of the dryer or the curling iron or something is usually necessary for a finished look.

If your hair is blown dry, watch again for evidences of real quality. A good style can't be even started until the hair is about 90 percent dry, but it makes a difference how you get to that point. Does the stylist let you sit around until your hair has begun to stick out in all its endearing little ways and then dry like crazy, trying to force it into a smooth line?

As you may have guessed, that's the wrong way. The right way is to blow the hair in the opposite direction from the way it lies until it's just slightly damp, then brush in the other direction to complete the style. If the stylist uses any conditioners or creams on your hair at this point, ask what they are and what they do. If you don't, you may find it impossible to duplicate the style at home, no matter how adept you are with the dryer and the brush.

SECOND DAY

Continue your diet, but don't step on the scales. This is important, so please don't cheat and sneak into the bathroom for a little peak. The psychological effects of weighing too much or too soon can be devastating. Follow your personal exercise routine, and don't forget to mark the chart.

Today we're going to talk about the hair you wish wasn't there at all—on your legs, under your arms, your upper lip, wherever. Unwanted hair is like noise—what bothers some people a lot is no problem at all for others. But I'd venture to say that even the fairest and most light-haired of us has at least some hair that has to be regularly removed or bleached or tweezed or something. It's a grooming task we all share, and this is the day you learn everything you're ever likely to need to know about it.

Shaving. This is what most of us do about most of our unwanted hair. It's a bit of a bore, but it's safe if you're careful, usually doesn't cause any skin irritation, and lasts, more or less, for a week. It's also the cheapest method of hair removal, and I recommend it for legs and underarms, also for the bikini line in the summer, though I wouldn't bother with this when it isn't going to show. (Some women say the same about legs, but I don't like trying to cut through that tangle when the day comes you want to get out of your long black cotton stockings.)

After shaving is an excellent time to apply a slightly abrasive dry-and-dead skin lotion to your legs to keep them from getting scaly looking. The lotion is also good for rough patches on heels, soles, elbows, and so forth. Or you may want to use pumice stone on the smaller areas, though I like the lotion for the whole job. If you use a chemical hair remover instead of shaving, wait a bit for the dead skin removal, since depilatories can irritate the skin somewhat more than shaving.

Bleaching. Bleaching is good for those areas where you simply can't afford any stubble—generally on the face, although some women bleach hair on the arms, belly, and other parts of the body. There's no reason those cream bleaches that work so well on your lip and chin won't work for hair on other parts of the body, too, though it may take more than one application and be a little inconvenient to lie around covered with bleach. The most common mistake in bleaching, from what I see around me, is leaving the bleach on too long. Instead of a dark mustache, the woman ends up with a mustache that's much lighter than all the rest of her facial hair, and stands out almost as much. You'll have to experiment with your favorite product to get the timing just right, but start with just a minute or two and work up. You can always scrape off the bleach and re-apply if the job needs more time.

Tweezing. This is what we do to the unwanted hairs that crop up more or less one at a time instead of in clumps. It usually means eyebrows, that one dark hair in your chin, the hairs at the fronts of your nostrils, and so on. If your mother used to tell you that plucking your eyebrows would make them grow in even bushier, relax: she was wrong. Habitual tweezing actually seems to have the opposite effect. If you were to stop, you'd probably find that your eyebrows grew in more sparse than before. That's something to consider when you decide just how thin a line to pluck. If fashions change, as they have a way of doing, you may be stuck with too thin an eyebrow if you've been plucking it that way for years. Keep to a moderate line, and you'll be more adaptable. Tweezing is one hair-removal practice that really has to be done every day to keep things smooth. It only takes a minute, since only a few hairs will be ready on any day, but if you let it go even a couple of days, you'll start to see stragglers. A few people would rather have the eyebrows bleached than tweeze them every day, but it's too risky to attempt this yourself, and costly in a salon.

Waxing. This is much less familiar to most of us, though it's been around a long time and can be done either by a salon professional or by you at home. The big drawback is that waxing hurts—it's a lot like removing a really stuck-on bandage. The big attraction is that hair stays away longer than with shaving or depilatories—up to six weeks between treatments on the legs, four weeks on the face. If you're thinking of switching to waxing, I suggest you make an appointment to have it done once in a salon before you undertake it at home. Any area of the body can have hair removed by waxing, but the most common are the upper lip, the legs, the bikini line, arms, and hands. Some women also wax off body hair, such as on the belly, or the hair under the arms—the tenderest area of all.

Essentially, what a wax treatment does is literally grab the hair and tear it out by the roots. Naturally, the skin usually reacts by turning red and swelling up a little. The reaction is usually over an hour or so after the treatment. In salons, where the operator has had lots and lots of practice, pain and the subsequent reaction is usually less severe.

For most women, the upper lip and the bikini line present the most sensitive excess-hair problems. The upper lip is so visible that any treatment that leaves or invites a five o'clock shadow is out of the question. The bikini line problem is one of sensitivity in the literal sense. The area may break out if shaved, waxed, or depilated. By the time the skin reaction is over, the hair is already growing back. As I've said, I think bleach is the answer for the lip, unless hair is so thick or so dark that it simply has to be removed. In that case, I'd say wax. As for the bikini line, my experience has been that good old-fashioned shaving works best here. Be sure there's a good, sharp blade in your razor, so you don't irritate the tender skin; then shave every day in the bathing suit season, during or right after your shower. Unless you're unusually thick-skinned, the bikini line isn't a good place to try waxing.

Permanent Hair Removal.   Unlike certain treatments for hair replacement, these are on the level. The older method is called electrolysis, and is only performed by salon professionals. The newer method is called Depilatron, and it, too, is available only in salons. Both work by destroying—hopefully for good—the center of the hair follicle. That way, no new hair can be produced. Electrolysis uses a needle that penetrates through the pore to apply heat to the papilla of the follicle. As you might suspect, the procedure can leave the skin red and needle-marked, especially if you've been worked on by a less-than-skilled practitioner. Marks usually go away, but once in a while there is permanent scarring. The other problem is that electrolysis can also be painful. The more sensitive the area from which hair is being removed, the more painful the process. Electrolysis works, however, which is its big plus. I would say that less is known about Depilatron, just because it hasn't been around as long as electrolysis. Since the newer process works with little electrified tweezers instead of little electrified needles, Depilatron doesn't hurt. Both Depilatron and electrolysis actually use shortwave radio waves to zap the hair follicles. But whereas the electrolysis needle has to touch the follicle directly, Depilatron works by sending the impulse along the hair and into the follicle. Can you be sure that after you go through all this the hair won't grow back? More sure with electrolysis than with Depilatron. But then again, electrolysis is much more uncomfortable. If you have facial hair in excess of most people or other hair problems that really bother you, you probably won't mind the expense or even the discomfort. But for ordinary amounts of facial hair and body hair, I think more ordinary methods are called for. Let me say that hair removal is a highly individual thing. I know a woman who has all the hair waxed off her face about every four weeks. All of it—eyebrows, peachfuzz on the cheeks, everything. She likes the nice, flat surface for application of makeup. Personally, though, I think it's too much trouble to go through to make your face into the perfect canvas.

THIRD DAY

Today is facial day. You may be used to going once a week to your favorite salon for a complete skin treatment, or you may be at the other extreme—a woman who has never had a facial in her life. Whichever describes you, you have something to learn. A salon facial is wonderful—pampering, relaxing, and great for the skin. But you can do some very interesting things at home, too, with common household ingredients and half the time. By all means have a professional give you a facial at least once, just so you can see what the treatment is like. But learn my Home Facial tricks, too.

Cleansing

Face cleaning doesn't mean soap. It's too drying. Oh, I don't say you must never use soap (a famous Hollywood star admitted to a magazine interviewer that she sometimes sneaks away and scrubs her face with good old soap, just for that irreplaceable squeaky-clean feeling). But you shouldn't use soap every time you wash your face, and you should never, never use anything except mildest baby soap. What to use all those other times? Here are a few ideas:

Oil: that's right, oil. It makes a wonderful cleanser, even for oily skin. If you have a highly refined cooking oil such as peanut or sesame, try one of those. Almond oil, from a good drug store, smells better than peanut or sesame, and you know fragrance adds to the luxury of it all.

Buttermilk: Delicious; if any happens to sneak into your mouth, no harm done. Buttermilk is especially good for skin with that winter-weary look—washed out and blotchy—or skin that tends to look muddy. If you have large pores or oily skin, mix a little table salt with the buttermilk for deep scrubbing.

Yogurt: plain, please. I've never seen the skin that can benefit from an application of jam or other flavorings.

Yogurt has a slightly astringent effect, good for normal-to-oily skin. If your skin is dry, and you can afford it, substitute sour cream or use the buttermilk cleanser.

Steaming

This is deep-pore cleaning, and it's a necessity for dry skins just as much as oily ones. Pores are opened by steaming and washed out by water vapor. Heat a large pot of water almost to boiling, then put the contents in a basin and cover with a towel. Now, lift the towel and sneak your head in under, being careful to keep the towel as well draped around the sink as you can so all the warmth doesn't escape. Don't put your face down too close to the hot water or you might burn your nose. This shouldn't be an uncomfortable process, but pleasant, warm, and steamy. Do it for 5-10 minutes, the longer the better, but don't put a crick in your back.

Washing

This is a kind of cleansing, too, the kind that comes after the steaming and floods the loosened dirt and oil out of the pores. The idea is to flush the face with lots of liquid. Best for this is a shower-head type sprayer—the kind that attaches to the sink and is supposed to be for washing your hair. But you can, if you want (shh) just splash lots of water on your face from a running faucet. If you want something a little nicer smelling than plain old tap water, mix about a tablespoon of lemon juice with 8 ounces of water. Put the mixture into a spray bottle and *spritz* it on your face. Whatever formula you use, it should be cold, and it should be done quickly as possible after the steaming. You don't want to give any new dirt time to settle into those opened pores.

Finger Stimulation

Massage is a well-known relaxant and circulation stimulator for almost every part of you except the face.

Yet the face is the part everyone looks at first. It's also the part that takes a continued beating from wind and weather—out in front in all seasons, taking the cold, the heat, the sun, everything. In a salon facial, I admit, the finger stimulations step is more relaxing than it can ever be at home, simply because you're doing it yourself at home. But you'd be surprised how relaxing it is, even to massage your own face. Begin by massaging about a tablespoon of the same oil cleanser you used to begin the facial. If you didn't use oil then, use it now—a good, clear oil—no face creams yet.

The Masque

This is the final essential pore-tightening step after the deep cleaning. If you aren't in the habit of giving yourself a frequent masque, you're missing one of the most effective ways to keep your skin looking fine-grained and flawless looking much longer than you would have thought possible. Keep in mind that the masque, just as cleaning, isn't a permanent tightening treatment. To achieve its long-range effects, it has to be used regularly. Many fine commercial masque preparations are on the market, or you can try one of these to whip up at home:

Milk masque. Pulverize one orange in your blender or food processor and add powdered milk until the mixture has a pasty consistency. For extra skin nourishment, drop in a 250 milligram vitamin C tablet. For dry skin, substitute a peeled cucumber for the orange.

Egg masque. Separate two eggs, saving the whites for cooking. Mix the two egg yokes with corn meal until the paste is the right consistency for a masque. If this mixture seems to harden too fast, add water by the drop to correct dryness.

Whatever masque you use, apply it to all areas of the face except the delicate area under the eyes and the lip area. (If you put it over your lips, you won't be table to talk as the mixture dries.) Leave on for ten minutes while you relax, preferably with eyes closed. Sponge off with cool water, dry your face, and apply your favorite moisturizer. Don't forget to take a good look in a magnifying mirror so you can see how really great your skin is capable of looking with proper attention.

FOURTH DAY

Check your exercise chart, and continue with your diet plan, but don't weigh in yet. Today is a good day to introduce variety into your diet plan. If you've been having cottage cheese for lunch all week, substitute another allowable protein food instead, for example, or have a big salad for dinner with cooked chicken instead of your usual beef.

Daily Treat

The Herbal Bath: Run the hottest bath your tub is capable of, and add to the water mint leaves (fresh or dried), pine needles, a spring of fresh basil or rosemary or, if all else is unavailable, a little powdered orange or lemon rind. If you don't like the idea of bathing in the same tub with bits of floating vegetation, tie the herbs in a cheesecloth bag, just like you do for the stew, and remove before you get in. The scented vapors are heavenly.

Mink Oil Bath: Remember mink oil? You can still get it, and it still works. This is an unjustly neglected beauty aid, in my opinion. Just a few drops in your bath will make you feel sleek as—well, as a mink.

Baking Soda Bath: A sure-fire old fashioned refresher. Just add a tablespoon or two of baking soda to the water before you get in. It's an all-over body skin conditioner and it just makes you feel so good.

Club Soda Rubdown: Mix in a tall glass, 1 part lemon juice to 2 parts club soda. It's really for splashing over your skin just before the final rinse, but you can also drink a little, should thirst get to you while you're in the bath.

Whiskey in the Tub: A friend of mine swears by this one, and even though it's not on the diet, I've included it for completeness. Try it after you get thin. Just take a jigger of whiskey, a jigger of lemon juice in which you've dissolved a suitable amount of sugar, mix them together in a glass, and take the whole concoction into the tub where you—yes, drink it. Slowly. While you steep. Not for every day, even when you're not dieting, but relaxing, for sure.

After the Bath: Splash on something cooling, pore-tightening. A good one to try is Sea Breeze antiseptic lotion. It's antiseptic because it contains alcohol—and that's why it's cooling, too. You don't have to have sunburn to use it.

FIFTH DAY

I hope you have a full day to devote to hair conditioners, but even if you don't, I've listed all the good ones for you to try. It's very helpful if you consider your bathroom a laboratory, if even for an hour, and actually experiment to see which preparation really does something for your hair. It's so much easier to know if you can compare one treatment to another on the same day. If you just can't see conditioning your hair so much in a single day, try the conditioners in sequence and jot down your reactions on a little chart so you can remember from session to session.

Mayonnaise Conditioner: Use the whole-egg kind, just as it comes from the jar, or make your own using 1 egg, 1 cup of oil, and a tablespoon of lemon juice. Apply the mixture, as much as you need, to your wet but unwashed hair and let it soak in for 10 minutes. Wash thoroughly until your hair squeaks. Plain old mayonnaise is good for your face, too—it's a marvelous combination of protein and fat. Just what skin and hair always needs.

Vaseline Conditioner: For really dry or damaged hair, this old home remedy can't be beat. It takes several shampooings to wash out, though, so don't make the mistake of once-over-lightly and expecting your hair to look lovely. You'll have to scrub more than usual after this treatment. Soften a few tablespoons of Vaseline over a double boiler and then combine with a teaspoon of Ivory Flakes. Mix together in a blender or with an electric beater until frothy and white. Use this like one of those deep conditioners that you put on your hair and leave for at least twenty minutes. For additional benefits, wrap a hot towel around your hair. As I said, you'll have to shampoo several times to get all the Vaseline out, but the results will be worth the effort.

Kelp Hair Bath: Combine milk powder and kelp powder (from the health-food store) with enough yogurt to make a workable paste. Apply to hair and let stand for 10 minutes, then shampoo. You won't believe the body this can give.

Henna: Yes, henna is for coloring your hair, but it's also a natural conditioner. Ask your beautician for the kind of henna conditioner that comes in capsules but adds no color to the hair, and follow the directions on the package. You won't see any change in hue, but oh the change in manageability. If you're like a lot of women I know, one trial will make you an addict.

SIXTH DAY

Diet: It's time to weigh in. If you've been restrained and haven't made any side trips to the scale before this, you should have a pleasant surprise in store for you. I can't emphasize enough how important it is not to step on the scale six times a day, or even once. A weighing a week is plenty. If you haven't lost at least two pounds, you're doing something wrong. Perhaps you need a diet scale to be sure you're not cheating on your portions. An ounce is probably less than you think.

Exercise: You should begin to see the results of my shape-up program. Your clothes—the very same ones—should fit better now over those trouble spots. Now may be the time to step up your fitness activities a bit, getting ready for your jump to the next level. Re-test whenever you think it's time.

Daily Treat

The Manicure: Second only to a beautiful face are beautiful hands. And it's the nails, as every women knows, that make or break the hands. Whether you have fabulous nails that seem to be made of plastic from Krypton, or whether you have nothing but bitten stubs, you can have lovely looking nails. Here's how.

1.   See a professional. If you have time and money enough, see her all the time. If not, go once and pick up all the tips you can, not to mention a set of handsome nails. Next time your manicure needs doing (in a week or so, usually), see if you can duplicate the procedure at home.

2.   Always soak before you manicure. First, remove all traces of old polish, then plunge your hands into a bowl or basin of mild, soapy water. (You can use dishwashing liquid just like the lady on the TV commercials, but be sure it's a mild one.)

3.   Dry hands and file nails into the shape you want. The shape I always want is a nearly perfect oval, just slightly flat at the top. I find this shape resists breakage the best. Use an emery board only. I've yet to meet the person who could do anything to nails with one of those metal files except tear them up. I think metal files are for prison bars, not fingernails.

4.   Use your favorite hand lotion, lavishly. If you have any dead or thoroughly roughened skin on your hands or around the nails, try a bit of the same foot-softening lotion you use after shaving your legs. This works especially well on the cuticles. After you've softened the cuticles, push them back with the blunt end of an orangewood stick. In salons, they cover the end of the

stick with cotton so there's no chance of bruising.

5. Clean under the tips of your newly-shaped nails with the sharper end of the orangewood stock. Again, use cotton for extra gentleness.

6. Apply a primer coat to the nails. Don't omit this step, even if you don't wear nail polish. It gives the nails a soft, clear shine and helps them resist breaking.

7. After the base coat, apply your color coats. How many applications you use depends on the kind and color of the nail polish, and also on the texture and length of your nails. The longer and tougher your nails are (or look), the stronger the color they can carry off.

Fabulous Fakes

Some women wouldn't be seen in public, ever, without a perfect set of nails. So what do they do when the garbage disposal eats up the prize Mandarin Forefinger Nail? They reach for one of the many kinds of acrylic fakes on the market, or perhaps for the phone to call the manicurist so that she can apply one of the acrylic fakes. Either way, the new plastic nails have caused a revolution in the hand business, and they make it possible for every woman to have perfect-looking nails all the time.

Since there is some trickiness involved in applying the fakes, and since they can actually make your own nails grow in deformed if they aren't done right, I do recommend that you see this done by someone who knows how before you try it on yourself. The main trick is not to completely cover the whole nail so that no air can reach down to your own finger. You'll avoid this if you use the fake kits exactly as directed, applying the acrylic liquid only around the edges and leaving your own nail room to breathe in the middle. When it's done skillfully and properly painted, you can't tell where your nail ends and the fake starts.

The Pedicure

How is it that so many people who have beautiful and

cared-for hands have feet they'd rather hide under a basket? Could it be they just haven't invested the time? Feet take a lot of abuse, of course, carrying the load of the whole body everywhere all day, and often doing it while crammed into ill-fitting shoes. But you don't have to have those horney calluses on your heels or those rough places on your ankle bones. And your toenails, believe it or not, can look as smooth and shapely as your fingernails do, if perhaps not so long and tempting.

The treatment for feet is essentially the same as for hands, except that you must soak your feet longer in soapy water. After the feet are dry, cut toenails straight across with a good sharp pair of scissors, then file for a smooth edge. You don't want to have the toenails rounded at all or you risk ingrown toenail, as painful a malady as it sounds. Don't use toenail clippers, either, it's a sure way to get ragged, uneven nails. Once the nails are done, apply a softening lotion to the feet. If you prefer, you can use pumice stone after the soaked feet are dry. It's available in all drug stores, and it works by sanding away the tough outer layer of dead skin on places like heels and the balls of the feet. I prefer the slightly abrasive foot lotions, however, because they work on the whole foot, including the area around the nails where you couldn't possibly use a pumice stone. Lotions smell nicer, too.

Once you've given your feet the treatment they deserve, you'll begin to see their natural beauty emerge. It's a fact that feet are much more sensual and sensuous than hands; the soles are just so sensitive. If you've never tried foot massage as a prelude to lovemaking, it's probably because you didn't think your feet would be attractive. Now that they are, ask your man to rub your feet for you, just once. I guarantee you'll never hold hands again.

SEVENTH DAY

This is the day to re-assess your exercise program. Are you finding jogging just too time-consuming and unpleasant? Maybe you should consider switching to jumping rope or running in place, both of which can be done indoors, provided you don't live in a top-floor apartment in a rickety building. A beautiful woman I know who lives in Toronto puts it this way, "Jogging? I love it. But not when the air outside is so cold that my nose feels like it's freezing every time I breathe in. That's why I always jog in place in my basement during the winter. You know what I do to keep it from getting too dull? I invite a friend over, and we do it together. You'd be surprised how fast the exercise period goes when there's somebody else there doing it too." On the other hand, maybe you've started out with rope-jumping and you find it insufferably boring. So why not get out along the jogging paths and see if you like it better? Remember, you can change exercise routines any time, as long as you pick equivalent activities.

Daily Treat

If you've been supposing you have to be a movie star or a big business mogul to have a health-giving, nerve-soothing massage once in a while, put the thought right out of your mind. It can't be denied that massage is at its best when it's done to a completely relaxed you by somebody else. That's so good, in fact, that it's worth going to some trouble to obtain: you might trade off massage sessions with your husband, for instance, or any other willing intimate friend. But there are times when there's nobody else available and you really need to do something to change your mood, iron a few of the wrinkles out of your psyche, and just generally get yourself up and ready to go out and face the world again. For those times, I want you to learn *self-massage*.

1. Relax all over. This is easier said than done, but there are plenty of time-tested techniques, and here's one: Lie on your back, eyes closed, and think about each part of your body in turn—your toes, your feet, your calves,

and on up. As you mentally focus on each set of muscles, consciously relax them, letting all tension drain away. When you get up to your shoulders, check to see that the legs haven't tensed up again. After a few practice sessions, you'll be able to keep yourself relaxed. I recommend you do this before massage to get the maximum benefit.

2. Elevate your legs and start your massage with the feet. I know you've probably seen massage done from the other direction, but I think the feet and legs need attention first. A good way to elevate the legs is to lie on the floor and prop your feet against the bed. Then reach up and start working your way up the feet and legs, pressing as hard as you like and moving your fingers in a circular pattern. (If you suffer from varicose veins or any kind of dermatitis, forget the massage. You can aggravate either condition by doing this.)

3. Do you want to use massage oil? Some people wouldn't consider leaving it out, while others feel using oil leaves the skin greasy. Actually, I'm of two minds. I do seem to finish up my oil massages with a bath, mostly because I feel over-oiled. But the stuff feels so wonderful while it's going on—much nicer than the same massage without oil. Perhaps the best solution is to bathe first, then use oil very lightly so that it's absorbed into the skin as the massage proceeds. Baby oil is my favorite—it's so light, and it smells good, too. On a cold day, or just because you want to, try heating the oil just a bit over hot water before you rub it into your skin.

4. You can massage your chest and arms in the same legs-elevated position, but you'll have to sit up to do a good job on your shoulders. Lean your back against the bed or wall, cross your arms, and work on each shoulder with the opposite hand. Try to relax everything except your hard-working fingers.

5. Finally, give those fingers a break. Massage each hand with the other, one at a time, and here's one place you don't have to skimp on the oil. Your fingers should

look pink (for a change) when you're through. That means you've got the blood flowing all the way up to the tips of your fingers again.

Head and Face

Face massage feels wonderful, but you must use cream or oil, otherwise you'll only be helping those little lines and wrinkles get a deeper hold on your visage. The best massage oil for the face is good old Vaseline. (I strongly suspect that someday it will be proven that Vaseline contains some secret ingredient that makes it superior to some of the most expensive creams, but it hasn't happened yet.) To make the Vaseline easier for the skin to absorb—so you won't look like you're greased up to swim the English Channel when you get done—heat a few tablespoons in the top of a double boiler until it melts. If you want to smell good, add a few drops of your favorite perfume. No scent clashes with Vaseline.

1. Massage the neck first, and always smoothe *downward.* (This may be contrary to what you've heard, but believe me, it's the right way. You won't do anything to counteract the effects of gravity with a few upward strokes, considering that gravity is at work twenty-four hours a day. All you'll do is help loosen the skin on your neck, making it more vulnerable to lines and wrinkles).

2. Do the cheeks next, with little semi-circular motions that move up and out, away from the mouth. The whole idea in a face massage is to smoothe the skin, not knead it.

3. Massage around the mouth, using long strokes that move up and out, toward the ears.

4. The forehead. A most important area for massage and for moisturizing, too. Use both hands, and start at a point just above the bridge of the nose, moving up and out in a pair of arcs that end at the temples. If you have deep frown lines, massage them separately, using two fingers in tiny, circular motions. I am firmly convinced that this is one area of wrinkling that responds very well

146

to massage.

5. The most natural thing to do when you've finished with your face is to move right on to a scalp massage. Unless your hair needs oil, be sure your fingers are clear of the Vaseline before you plunge into the hair. Begin at the temples, massaging in little circles that gradually get larger as you feel your scalp loosening. As you may know, the scalp is quite loose on the skull, and if you're applying enough pressure and your face is relaxed, you can feel the scalp move back and forth as you massage. Now move up and back with both hands, using either the same circular motions or a back-and-forth massage, whichever feels better to you. When your hands come together at the top back of your head, proceed to the top of your skull. Last, but most important, is the lower skull and the back of the neck. When you've done this, you'll have a strong desire to start the whole process all over again with the shoulder-massage. If you have time, go ahead. Otherwise, end your session with another minute or so of all-over relaxation, and head for the shower. The personal massage is a present you can give yourself any time you need a lift and there's nobody around to help but yourself.

EIGHTH DAY

Wardrobe Day. If you're starting to see the results of your exercise and diet programs by now—as you should if you've been faithful—this will be a treat for you. You're going to pull all those shirts and pants and dresses and sweaters and odds and ends out of the closet and try to make some sense of them in terms of wardrobe planning. Depending on how many clothes you've collected, this will take at least two or three hours, maybe more. If you can't fit it all into one day, use two, but don't put it off until next week, or you won't ever get the whole job done.

If you're like a lot of women, you have many more clothes than you ever wear. Why is that? Usually, it's because the clothes don't fit. Either they don't fit you, or they don't fit the fashion image you want to project, or they don't fit with each other. On this day of your 14-Day Makeover, you're going to assess all the clothes in your closet to see if they fit, and if not, why not. You're going to be ruthless in getting rid of clothes that absolutely won't do, but you're also going to discover some uses for clothes you thought were finished as working pieces of your wardrobe. After today, if you hear yourself crying that you have "nothing to wear," at least you'll know why.

Before you take inventory of the closet, take inventory of yourself. Do you know your fashion type? Your figure strengths and weaknesses? Basically, there are two fashion types. If you've never made up your mind which one is you, that could explain the muddle you find when you open the drawers. There's the Classicist, and there's the Modern. The Classicist doesn't follow the trends so much as she follows her own sense of what kinds of clothes will last. The Modern knows how to look up-to-the-minute by buying just a few pieces every so often that lend the latest look to her whole collection. The Classicist buys fewer clothes, shops less, follows fashion trends less. She may have to pay more for each individual piece, since she's buying for the long run, but she probably allocates less of her total budget for clothing than does the Modern. The Modern is the sort of woman who can't keep her eyes off the fashion pages, even when she wants to. She can hardly help passing through the department store on her lunch hour. Shopping is a pleasure to the Modern, something of a burden to the Classicist. Models, fashion editors, most people involved in the clothing business in any way and most celebrities are Moderns. Business women, teachers, scientists and medical workers tend to be Classicists. Curiously, visual artists, such as painters, may be either Classicists or Moderns, depending on whether they look on their clothes as objects of artistic attention or objects of functional utility. Novelists and poets are almost always classicists.

Which fashion type is yours? Give it some thought. Many of us had mothers who were Classicists, and tried to bring us up that way, too. That doesn't mean you have to stay in the mold, now that you're a grownup. On the other hand, you needn't feel a moment of guilt if you don't like to follow the trends and never will. The important thing isn't which type you are, but knowing it. Then you can plan a wardrobe that will really reflect you and your lifestyle. If you have trouble, consider whether you'd rather go downtown and look for a new dress or curl up with a good book. Do you hate it when a trusted piece of clothing wears out, or does it make you happy because now you can buy something more stylish? Questions like these are more important than whether you like or dislike any current look. If you're a true Modern, you can adapt any style to your personal tastes, and if you're a true Classicst, you really like your basic look to stay the same through the years, updated just enough with new accessories, different lengths, perhaps a few alterations. (The majority of men are Classicists, by the way, but that doesn't mean you have to go in for the Menswear look if you find yourself in that category.)

Now, for your figure. No matter what your fashion type, there's a way to dress to emphasize your strong points and camouflage your weak ones. If you think about it, you probably know all about your figure already. Is your head large or small? Is your neck long? Short? Wide or narrow shoulders? Big bust? Small bust? High or thick waist? Hips too big, or maybe you have a flat bottom? Most of us need to lose a few pounds, which is why your makeover includes my diet. But only you and your doctor know just how much you need to lose. Diet and exercise are busy shaping up your figure, but you can put your clothes to work to minimize your figure faults in the meantime.

Whatever your figure type, clothes that are too tight will only emphasize the flaws. As you go through your wardrobe, trying on absolutely everything, please, make a separate pile for those things that just don't seem to stretch across all of you. As your weight goes down, you can return to this pile. Don't discard anything yet, until you see how it fits when it *fits*. Most clothes look better when they're slightly loose, so don't throw away any of the items that you just "know" are too large—not until you try them on. And don't forget to mix and match. The idea of Wardrobe Day is for you to put all your clothes together in every conceivable outfit. You'll be surprised at least once or twice when some piece you were sure was worthless suddenly blossoms in tandem with just the right skirt or pair of pants. Don't forget your accessories in this orgy of try-ons. A dress that seems too plain for words without your gold chains might become very witty with the right extra touches.

The basic things to watch for as you go through your collection are these: Interchangeability. One reason you may have so many clothes and nothing to wear is that the clothes don't go with each other. On the other hand, maybe they do go together, but you just haven't made the connections yet. Color: If you're basically a modern, you probably have too much un-coordinated color. If you're a Classicist, you'll tend to have too little. Make plans now to buy one or two new pieces that will tie it all together. (Color is another good way to diagnose your fashion type. The Classicist tends to love one or two colors, year in and year out. The bulk of her wardrobe will be in classic neutrals that partner the colors—greys, black, beige, brown. The Modern is always interested in what's new in color and what she has that will go with it.) Style: This is the most subtle factor, but probably the most important. If you're a tailored type, it's easy to see why that expensive ruffled print dress never gets any wear. But if you're only comfortable in very feminine clothes, there's no use buying this year's blazer and jeans just to be in the mode. You'll always feel like you're impersonating a boy when you wear the outfit. And don't forget that if you like to wear your hair very short, you'll have to balance that look with feminine clothes and suitable makeup, or you really will look like a boy. If you like your clothes very tailored, you might consider at least a medium-length hairstyle.

NINTH DAY

This is the day you analyze your hair and plan a program of regular care. To begin with, take a good look in the mirror at your new haircut. You must have washed your hair at least once by now—so how does the haircut look? Does it resemble the way it looked when you walked out of the salon, or does it look more like it did when you walked in? Are you happy about that, or not? Assuming you had a first-class haircut (a must), the one-week later test tells more about you than about your stylist. If you've been able to maintain the look the stylist gave you, it's probably because the look suits you and the amount of work you're willing to put in on your hair. If not, maybe you should be more emphatic next time in asking for a style you can do yourself. Be willing to admit to the stylist what you can and can't do in the way of setting, blow-drying, and so on.

If you're having trouble maintaining a look you really want, let's see if we can find out why. Short hair styles have to be washed every day, and it has to be in the morning, because sleeping all night on your hair tends to bend it in funny ways, even if it's clean. Are you willing or able to do that? Oily hair has to be washed just about every day, too, so short hair goes well with this type. Since you have to wash anyway, you might as well have less hair to wash and less drying time, right? Long styles, which keep their shape through nights of tossing and turning because of the weight of the hair, are best for normal-to-dry hair. That way, if you miss one shampoo day, you won't look like an oil-drenched cocker spaniel the next day. This isn't to say that if you have oily hair, fine hair, thin hair, or all three that you can never wear an over-the-ears style. It'll just be more work for you. The question here is one of lifestyle. Are you organized enough to put in the time? Do you want to? Remember, you can't have both wash-and-wear hair and the look that duplicates that of your favorite star. Not unless your hair is a duplicate of hers and *she* has wash-and-wear hair—an unlikely event.

What about conditioning? The more chemical treatment you subject your hair to, the more compensating conditioning it will need. Before you color or permanent, remember that it's a commitment to more than just color or curls. After the treatment, it will take you more time and more hair-care products to keep your hair in the same condition it used to be in with no time or trouble at all. Is it worth it to you to have a livelier color or more body in your hair? For lots of women, the answer is an emphatic "yes!" But you don't have to act like lots of women. If you'd rather be gray and not have to spend all that time massaging conditioners into your hair, then that's your choice. Gray hair can be very attractive, especially when it's complemented by pretty colors near the face, a young hairstyle, an active body. If you work it right, nobody will think of you as gray without adding the word "premature."

How well do you handle the styling end of your hairstyle? If it requires a blow-dryer to get the look you like, can you do the job yourself? Do you have the kind of hair that will hold a blown-dry style, or does it really need a firmer set to stay in shape all day? One of the most blessed trends in hairstyling today is the move toward styles suited for types of hair rather than to the iron demands of this year's clothes. Be realistic about your hair type as well as about yourself and your abilities as a stylist. If your hair's straight as a pin and won't curl unless you sleep on rollers all night, why not just give up and wear your hair straight? Some of your curly-haired sisters would give anything for the kind of sheen that only shows on straight hair. And if the Afro's the only cut your hair can keep without steam pressing, why not? Are you aware of how many women are paying fortunes for curly perms these days? It may be easier to unload your preconceptions about perfect beauty than to change your hair.

Standard Oily Hair Routine

1. Wash at the first sign of greasiness. For most, that means every day. If your hair's thick-textured, it may withstand the greasies for two days. If it lasts more than that, it's not what I'd call oily hair. Use a conditioning shampoo specially formulated for hair that's washed often.

2. Condition once a week. Since you have the kind of hair that can't stand creme rinse, you must use the kind of conditioner that washes out after application. In the winter, when the air's dryer and your hair's less oily, "instant conditioner" may help.

3. Haircut every six weeks without fail. Oily hair grows faster than other kinds, maybe because the same mechanism that produces too much oil also aids growth. If you wear bangs, you may have to have your hair cut every four weeks to keep them from turning into greasy strings in your eyes.

4. Electric curling irons, blow-dryers and electric curlers were made for you. Your hair can stand up to them better than any other type. Since you have to wash your hair often, why not do it in the mornings and finish quickly with electric beauty aids? Your style's at its loveliest when you haven't slept on it.

Standard Dry Hair Routine

1. Establish a washing schedule. You'll know how often your hair needs washing by the way it looks. When hair

starts to go dull and the style starts to sag, it's time to reach for the shampoo. For most people with dry hair, twice a week is enough to wash, and for some it's once a week. Whenever you wash, be sure you allow plenty of time for:

2. Conditioning. Most people with your hair type need both a deep conditioner regularly and a rinse after shampooing to put back the shine that detergent takes away.

3. Be sure to get a cut suited to your hair type. If your hair's fine, only a good blunt cut will prevent it from flying away, especially in the winter. If your hair's heavy, you can wear one of the longer, swinging styles. Just be sure to have it trimmed every six weeks to two months so that the line stays clean. If you happen to be blessed with heavy, dry, and curly hair (think Gilda Radner) you can wear one of those gloriously frizzy halos that seems to go on forever. Cute.

4. If you use electric appliances, use a conditioner especially formulated to protect your hair from the drying effects. This goes double if you color or perm. Good for dry hair are the kinds of conditioners you massage in just before drying—you don't rinse them out at all, yet they don't grease down your hair.

TENTH DAY

This is the first day of your makeup planning Makeover, which will consume the remainder of the week. Don't forget to exercise, and stick to your diet, but don't weigh in. That won't come until Day 14.

If you've been into a department store or cosmetic specialty store lately, you may have been bewildered by what's available. You may even have collected a surplus of little tubes and jars, and find them littering your dressing table or bathroom without doing a single thing for your face. On this day I'll tell you which products you need, and which you can pass by.

Tools

You'll need cotton balls or squares, a set of little sponges, tissues, and eyelash curler if you like. (I don't use one because I find it tends to make my lashes break off—most undesirable.)

Pencils, if you prefer them to creams. Available are lip pencils, eyeliner and eyeshadow pencils.

Brushes—the major makeup tools. Two large, soft paintbrushes, one for powder and one for blusher. An eyeshadow brush for every color you use. Children's toothbrushes, one for the brows and one for the lashes. Eyeliner and lip brushes if you don't use pencils.

Basic Makeup Products

Most people need most of these. We'll discuss the specific types when we talk about eyes, lips, and face shaping, but this is what should be in your makeup kit or at least standing at the ready in the medicine cabinet.

Cleansers
Makeup removing products
Skin freshener and/or astringent
Blemish and antiseptic treatment products
Foundation
Cover-up stick
Blushers and contouring products
Eyeliner
Eye shadow
Mascara
Lip colors and glosses
Powder (if you like it)

ELEVENTH DAY

We devote the makeover time on this day to your eyes. Time after time in salon makeovers, these are the points that seem to crop up:

* Bushy Brows. Most of us start out with a fairly natu-

ral look when we're young, and that's fine. But the brows tend to droop a bit as time goes by, so that older women look better with less brow than they had when younger. One problem with brow shaping seems to be that women just don't know where or how much to pluck. My advice: have it done professionally once, then follow the line. Basically, eyebrows should start just above the inner corner of your eyes—a bit further back if you have close-set eyes. The arch should be gentle and natural, with no stragglers between brow and eyelid. If you haven't been plucking enough, don't start yanking the hairs out in clumps. Pluck one hair at a time, working upward from the bottom. Once you have the shape you like, tend to it *every* day, so it never gets out of shape again.

* If your brows are very dark, you'll want to make them even thinner. Instead of pencil or other color, use your coverup stick lightly on the brows at makeup time, then brush them into place with a toothbrush. The coverup will lighten the brows slightly and it's sticky enough to keep them in place.

* Do not use face bleach on your eyebrows. Don't use haircolor, either. You could permanently damage your eyes at worst. At best, you'll end up with orange eyebrows or brows that look like they belong on the face of a movie surfer.

* Eyeliner has been out of fashion for a while, but not with me. The soft pencils give color and definition without seeming harsh, and I've never seen the eye that didn't look better with a touch of liner. If you're dark, choose brown or black. For blondes, gray and taupe are best. Never use bright jewel colors, either on lids or for liner.

* Nothing looks worse than eye makeup that has run into the wrinkles around your eyes. Moisturizer around the eyes helps the wrinkles, but it also encourages smearing. If your skin is oily or if you wear extra moisturizer around the eyes, use a powder eyeshadow and 24-hour mascara. Even then, use it lightly and check it often in a

mirror. Better to de-emphasize your eyes a bit than to look like you've literally cried your eyes out.

* The darker your skin, the brighter the color you can get away with on the lids. For pale skin, bright blue, plum, green, purple, all seem to draw attention away from your eyes and toward the color you've painted the lid. Whatever color you use, use a slightly darker version in the crease.

* Use face powder, even if you don't use it for anything else, to powder your lashes before you put on your mascara. And use a brush afterwards so that your lashes won't look like gunked-up spider's legs. Unless you've had exceptional good luck with it, don't mascara your lower lashes. For most people, the color soon ends up in a ring beneath the eye.

* Your coverup stick is the best tool for contouring eyes. White under the eyes (and between them if your eyes are close together) often gives a surprising bull's eye effect—not what you want at all. No matter what color coverup you use on the rest of your face, use light under your eyes.

TWELFTH DAY

Diet: If you think you're doing well, you may weigh in early today. If you have some catching up to do, wait until Day 14. Remember that all is not lost if you exceed your allowance on any one day. Dieting is for the long term, and the important thing is to have your caloric intake average the right amount over the week. The last two days are a good time to make up for minor sins.

Daily Treat

Facial contouring is a model's trick that too many of us don't know anything about. I've seen women who were absolute wizards on their eyes, but didn't use so much as a touch of blusher on the cheeks. This makes for an unbalanced, overly pale look—rather stark. The more eye makeup you wear, the more important it is to balance it on cheeks and lips. Blushers and contour (brownish) colors come in powder, creme and pencil form. If your skin's oily, you'll probably like the powder. If it's dry or lined, stick to pencil or creme.

Cheek color is for making your cheekbones stand out. The idea is to enhance and even out the natural color that almost everybody has in the cheeks. If you can't see any in yours, go outside on a nippy day, or check your face after your exercise period when you've been breathing hard. Where the color is naturally is the same place you want to put it with art—only just a bit more. If you feel your face is too florid, use a light color only to even your own coloring. If your face is pale, deepen your color a bit and extend it out, away from the nose, to cover slightly more area. Notice, I said slightly more. You don't want to end up looking like a kewpie doll.

Contouring is done to shape the face rather than to highlight any particular area. The commonest places for contouring color are just under the cheeks, along the nose, and under the chin. Experiment with brownish contouring color, remembering that the basic principle is: if you want to emphasize a feature, make it lighter. If you want to de-emphasize it, make it darker. That means that contouring color would be good for that bump on your nose, to minimize it just a bit, and for your double chin. Be sure that the color's well-blended so you don't look hastily stripped instead of shaped.

THIRTEENTH DAY

Unlucky thirteen—but not today. Today you work on your mouth, a much-neglected area of late when it comes to makeup. The big problem: lip color can look harsh, and it can fade. The big plus: next to the eyes, lips are everybody's best feature. Most people look at your mouth when you talk to them, even more than at your eyes. And lip color can correct such a multitude of flaws. If you haven't worn any lipstick but California pale for ten years, now's the time to bring your lip routine up to date.

A Short History of Lipstick

Once upon a time, perhaps when your mother was a young woman, a grownup female wouldn't be caught dead in public without her lipstick. Eye makeup was in its infancy then, except for actresses, and most women wore nothing, except maybe eyebrow color. As women began to emphasize their eyes more and more, lip color seemed to fade out of fashion. There was a time, and most of us remember it, when *the* look was huge, black-lined eyes and no color on the lips at all. Some women even tried to make their lips paler by using white lipstick. Finally, it dawned on women that the look was a little bit sickly, and lip color began to make a cautious comeback. The first products to win wide acceptance among the young were lip glosses—a little color and a lot of slickness. Glosses were good for the lips, too, which need almost constant protection in every season if they aren't going to chap and peel. Gradually, women discovered again that lip color made their whole face look better. Now, most of us wouldn't go out of the house without at least a shiner and a hint of color.

Here's what you need for the well-dressed mouth:
gloss
lipstick (the real thing)
lip pencils
brushes

The pros and cons: *Gloss* goes on easily, has a natural, see-through color, and makes your mouth look shiny and sexy. Unfortunately, gloss also comes off easily, so that most of us have trouble keeping any color on more than a few minutes. Unless you want to apply lip color every few minutes, you need a more stable color for the base, gloss for highlighting and brightening the color.

Lipstick has deeper color and more wax for longer lasting

cling. For some, the colors just as they come from the tube are too intense, but a happy medium can be achieved by first applying lipstick, then blotting, then finishing with a dab or two of gloss.

Lip pencils are for lining the lips. This is especially important if there are lines around your mouth into which lipstick tends to run, or if you're trying to correct your mouth shape with coloring agents. Lip liner keeps color where you want it, and away from where you don't.

For application of lipstick proper, a lip brush is essential. If you try to apply straight from the tube, you'll get a blurred line at best, an off-center smear if you're not so lucky. Defects of mouth shape and balance of lips can be corrected by lining the color either slightly outside or slightly inside your natural lip line. Fill in with a slightly lighter color, blend, and apply a bit of gloss over the top. Don't try to drastically re-shape your mouth, however. The illusion only works if the drawn line is very close to the natural one. Otherwise, it just looks as though you applied your lipstick in the dark. A trick models use that works very well for the rest of us is to make the lip you want to emphasize a bit darker than the other one. (This is an exception to the rule that darker-colored areas tend to recede.)

FOURTEENTH DAY

Diet: It's weigh-in time for everyone. If you've followed my diet, you should be four to seven pounds lighter, and your clothes should show the change. If you've been following your personal exercise program, the pounds will seem really to have melted off, with no tell-tale sagging skin left behind. It's really amazing how much thinner you can be in just two weeks, especially after trying unsuccessfully to lose over long periods on what I call "yo-yo" diets. (Drastic downs followed quickly by drastic ups.)

The last day of your Makeover is set aside for establishing a makeup routine, similar to your hair-care routine, your diet routine, your exercise routine. The idea of the Makeover, you see, is to help you set up new habits that will persist long after you've finished reading this book. The lower limit for a complete daily makeup seems to be about ten minutes. I know women who've been trying to shave seconds off that time for years, but savings so far haven't been significant. Ten minutes in the morning is ten precious minutes, but since it sets your look for the whole day, it's worth it. This is the standard routine:

1. Moisturizer. This is most effective if it's applied directly to a well washed face. What you want to do is trap moisture on the skin with a thin film of oil. Use your favorite product, whatever seems to work best for you, but apply it liberally, to temples and neck as well as to the face.

2. Foundation. The purpose of foundation is to even out your skin tone and cover tiny flaws. The kind you choose will depend on your particular skin and what kind of shape it's in. If you have lines and wrinkles, use one of the new, airy souffle foundations, and don't use much. If you have blemishes to cover, first apply a medicated ointment, then perhaps one of the heavier-coverage foundations. If you have good skin, don't skip this step, just buy one of the clear, natural foundations that impart no color of their own, but just even out yours. Remember, foundation tends to collect in wrinkles and scars, so don't overdue it around these areas.

3. Coverup stick. This is a heavier face color, mixed in a base of wax for maximum sticking power. It's too heavy for over-all face color, but perfect for erasing little blemishes, freckles, shadows, and lines. If you have deep wrinkles, don't fill in with makeup, as it will only make you look like your face is cracking.

4. Cheek color and contouring: Don't try either of these

techniques for the first time during a ten-minute morning session. Practice first, when you have plenty of time, until you can do what needs to be done without thinking. If you use liquid color, dot and blend. If you use powder, be sure it shades gradually into the rest of your makeup.

5. Eyes: Here's how I do it: eyeliner first, put on in little dots (or dashes if you use a pencil), then blended for a slightly smudgy line. Eyeshadow next, further blending the line over the eye and darker in the crease. A touch of powder on the lashes, then mascara. If you want to curl your eyelashes, do it before applying the powder.

6. Lips: Liner first, a nice, clean, easy to see pencil line. Then fill in with lipstick color and finish with a dab of gloss, just in the center of your mouth. If lipstick color's too intense, blot before you apply the gloss coat.

7. Finish: Most women like to blot the entire face a bit to take the "done" look off and avoid a mask-like appearance. Depending on your face type, you could use a bit of moisturizer on a cotton square, or just cool water. If you have a fine mist sprayer, it's perfect for "setting" your ten-minute face. Just fill it with cool water and spray ever-so-lightly, just as though you'd walked through a foggy morning.

QUESTIONS AND ANSWERS

Q: I've been trying everything to try to reduce my round tummy, but it stays round. Is it possible I'm just built that way, and exercise can't help?

A: No, it's not. Some people do have a greater tendency to collect fat in one place or another, or to get out of shape quicker in certain spots. But exercise can always help if you do the right ones the right number of times. The best one for flattening the stomach is the leg lift, and you have to do it a lot—as many as a hundred times a day. Always lift your head when you do this one so you won't strain your back. You may also need to lose a few pounds, and exercise will make sure you lose them where you want to.

Q: Do these new wrinkle-tamer lotions I've read about really work?

A: Yes, but only temporarily. After you put them on, your skin will look smoother, the wrinkles less pronounced, but the effect only lasts a few hours. Please understand that such lotions don't do anything to the wrinkles except make them appear less pronounced.

Underneath it all the wrinkles are there, unchanged.

Q: Can anything be done about little red spidery blotches on the face?

A: Yes, they can be faded in various ways by a dermatologist. But wait a little before you rush off to seek medical advice. Often, these broken capillaries fade of their own accord—a less painful and costly process.

Q: Are you opposed to high-heeled shoes?

A: That's a tough question. For occasional fashion punch, high heels are a must. But for daily wear, I guess my training as an exercise teacher has to win out. High heels throw your body off balance and don't permit full use of the muscles of your legs. When I see a teen-aged girl tip toeing around on four-inch heels, I imagine how she's going to be hobbling in the years to come from atrophied calf muscles. Think of it this way: your feet take a beating as it is, carrying all the load by themselves. How much more unfair is it to put all your weight on just half the foot?

Q: I seem to have a backache all the time. Could exercise help?

A: It could, if your lower back pain is due to poor muscle tone. But since so many other things can also cause backache, and a few of them can be made worse by the wrong kinds of exercise, see your doctor first.

Q: How much exercise is enough to keep fit?

A: It depends on who you are. Professional football players need about six hours a day or the muscle starts to turn into fat. For most of us, 30 to 60 minutes a day is about right, but that doesn't mean you have to devote an hour a day to pushups. A brisk half-hour walk is one of the best exercises I know.

Q: Is dancing good exercise?

A: Again, it depends. The foxtrot, no. The hustle, maybe. A half hour ballet class, definitely. You have to be exercising heavily enough to increase your heart rate and, pardon me, to sweat.

Q: What do you think about wigs?

A: Basically, they're still for the stage. A lot of women, including me, went through a phase when we thought wigs were going to be the answer to the frizzies, the greasies, the droopies, and just about every other hair problem. Hair didn't look so hot—just pop on a wig. But wigs just don't look natural enough for most of us. I'd say they're still good for emergency use, if you get a good one. Switches and hair pieces, to mix with your own (long) hair will have a lot of potential.

Q: If I had to buy one wardrobe item, starting from scratch, what should it be?

A: A good, really good, black wool skirt. If you wear pants most of the time, you might want to substitute a good, really good, pair of black wool pants. If fortune should smile on you and let you buy two items, number two should be a black velvet jacket.

Q: Will gelatin help my hair and nails grow longer?

A: To be blunt, no, it won't. The rationale of that old saw is that gelatin is almost pure protein, and so are hair and nails. Unfortunately, the protein in gelatin isn't a very useful one for the human body, and your hair and nails will continue to be made of protein, whether it comes in as milk, meat, eggs, or baked beans. A severe protein deficiency could hurt your hair and nails, but if you ever suffer from such a serious problem, hair and nails will be the least of your worries.

Q: Is it ever permissible to squeeze blackheads?

A: Squeeze is the wrong word. There are times when the most patient of us can't wait for nature to ever so gently wash away skin impurities, and we just have to give her a little help. If you must, here's how: first, steam clean your face according to the procedure you've already learned. Then, with fingers swathed in tissue, gently press the skin on either side of the blackhead. If your oil clog won't budge with such indirect treatment, give up and wait until it loosens up. Once you've got to the point of digging into the skin with your fingernails, you're doing much more damage and making your skin look much worse than a single blackhead. And remember, blackheads don't leave scars, but picking does.

Q: Is very pale skin a sign of ill health?

A: Usually, it's just a sign of a person's having inherited very pale skin. In the absence of other symptoms, it's probable that there's nothing wrong with your health, no matter how pale you may be. If you get tired of hearing people call you "poor pale Pam," work out a new makeup routine that adds more color via foundation, cheek color, and contouring. Don't try to bake yourself in the sun all the time to get a "healthy" look, or they'll soon be calling you "poor *old* Pam."

Q: Every time I color my hair, it smells bad for several days. I don't know if anyone else notices, but I sure do. Is there anything I can do about this?

A: Any of the scented creme rinses or instant conditioners will help take the "processed" odor away, as well as helping the texture of your hair. If it's still there, next time try a tomato-juice rinse. That's an old remedy for taking skunk odor off of dogs, and if you don't mind the backwoods connotations, it works for synthetic odors, too.

Q: I know you don't advocate crash diets, but what if I just have to lose a quick five pounds to fit into my new dress? Isn't there some diet I can follow, just for a week?

A: Depending on how heavy you are, it is possible to lose five pounds in a week. The loss will be mostly water, and it will come back in a single day if you go back to your old eating habits. If your livelihood depends on being able to squeeze into a dress, you might try a strict high-protein diet such as Dr. Stillman's—no fat, no carbohydrates. Don't stay on it more than a week, and don't forget to take your vitamins. When the week is over, switch to my Makeover diet for lasting weight loss.

Q: I have only a few gray hairs, but it seems to me they're coming in coarse and curly. Since my hair has always been fine and straight, I find it hard to believe. Is it possible?

A: Not only possible, but very likely. Gray hair has a different texture—sometimes very different from your younger hair. Some women find the renewed body (or coarseness, as you call it) a blessing, but some are annoyed at the way the gray hairs won't lie smoothly with the others. While you have only a touch of gray, it won't be much trouble to blend it in. As more of your hair changes in color and texture, you might want to consider a new hairstyle that takes into account the behavior of your new hair. (Coloring, by the way, won't alter the fact that your gray hair has a different texture.)

Q: I am two entirely different sizes, depending on the time of the month. Will taking diuretics help me shed some of the excess water I seem to hold?

A: It might, but it might also be bad for your kidneys. Don't take diuretics except on a doctor's advice. If you suffer from periodic bloating, keep your weight where it should be, and keep a few looser clothes for the bad days. It's better than tampering with your body's internal economy just for the sake of your tight-fitting jeans.

Q: Isn't there any place I can go to have the bulges just jiggled off by machine? I've seen so many interesting devices in ads for gyms and health clubs.

A: Not the good health clubs. In my clubs, there are no machines for "jiggling it off." The plain fact is that exercise is work. If you don't use the muscles, they won't build up, and the fat won't go away. You might find it pleasant to be bounced around in some sort of gimmicky machine, but don't fool yourself that it's helping to re-shape your body, anymore than the Ferris Wheel does.

Q: What can I do about the folds of loose skin that seem to be collecting as I get thinner?

A: First, exercise. As your muscles develop, they'll take up the space left by the water and fat you've lost. Second, massage. Give yourself a body rub every day with moisturizing lotion to help skin stay supple and smooth. Third, *gradual* weight loss, the healthiest way, is also best for preventing the Basset Hound Droop. Give your skin a chance to adapt to the reduced size of the body it's covering.

Q: I had a nose job when I was sixteen, which I now realize was too early. The perky little nose that looked so great at the Junior Prom just doesn't fit my grownup face. Is there anything that can be done?

A: Yes. See the same plastic surgeon who did your nose the first time and tell him or her the problem. Lucky for you, rhinoplasty leaves no visible scars, so nose jobs can be done twice or even three times without making you looked stitched together. Be sure you're not just "moving the furniture," though, for lack of something better to do.

Q: I'm not in high school, but sometimes my skin still looks like it. Should I use the same medicated pads I used then, or is there something better?

A: Adult skin can still suffer breakouts, but it can't take the rough treatment some adolescent girls give their skin. Most teenage blemish lotions are too drying for anyone over twenty-five. For my money, the best blemish treatment is a good cleansing with your regular gentle cleansing product, followed by a dab of anti-bacterial ointment such as you probably keep around for cuts and scratches. This can be spread thin to go under makeup where it stays all day to help heal and prevent infection. If you suffer more than periodic patches, consult a dermatologist.

Q: Don't you have anything to recommend for cellulite?

A: Nothing that I don't recommend for shaping and toning the body—diet and exercise. Cellulite, though it may look different from other kinds of subcutaneous fat, is really the same stuff. The only way to get rid of it for good is through diet and a program of regular exercises. If you are especially troubled by fat on the insides of your thighs, step up the number of one-leg lifts—the kind where you lie on your side and lift the top leg straight up. Walking, with long, long strides, is also especially good for heavy thighs.

Q: You may not believe this, but I'm too busy chasing after my four young sons and cleaning house to get enough exercise. I'm thin enough, but I know I'm out of shape. What do you suggest?

A: You're right, I don't believe it. I'm a mother of sons myself, so I know they can be a handful. But I also know there's time in the busiest of days for a moderate amount of exercise. Why don't you include the boys, if they're old enough, in a jumprope routine? Jumping isn't only for girls, you know, just ask Muhammed Ali. If your house has stairs, put them to use in your fitness program. Running up and down the stairs for five or ten minutes is strenuous enough for any athlete, and you don't even have to stop to pick up a rope. If you think that sets a bad example for the kids, do it when they're asleep. Or why not get involved in games with the kids? With your family, you've got an instant basketball team.

Q: My biggest beauty problem is my double chin. I'm not fat anywhere else, so what can I do?

A: First, check your posture. You might not have a double chin if you sat up straight and held your head erect. If that's not the problem, try this facial exercise ten times a day: stick your chin forward as far as it will go and say "eeee," very hard. If you're doing it right, the cords in your neck should stand out. (You don't have to say anything aloud, actually, just look as if you are.) The right look is something like an enraged monkey, but it really helps. Don't wrinkle up your brow while you do this, or you'll end up trading your double chin for a furrowed forehead.

Q: My makeup always seems to dissolve as the day goes by. Aren't there any products that don't require continual touch-ups?

A: The cosmetic industry is aware of our needs, and they're working on it. I predict major breakthroughs in the staying power of makeup—all kinds—in the next few years. In the meantime, carry a touch-up kit with you, consisting of a small tube of foundation, your coverup stick, lipstick, and mascara. For quick cleansing, a miniature bottle of baby oil and some cotton puffs.